The
Neuropsychologist's
Workbook

Drs. Hickle and Block are experienced neuropsychologists with a passion for mentoring emerging neuropsychologists. This workbook combines real-world advice, actionable strategies, and inspiring tips to empower you on the path to becoming a board-certified neuropsychologist. There is no roadmap like this.

—**Marc A. Norman, PhD,** University of California, San Diego

This book pulls back the curtain as to how to pursue a career in clinical neuropsychology, from start to finish. For the first time, aspiring and current students have a comprehensive go-to resource that provides clear and practical hands-on tools, coupled with sound advice from recognized experts in education and training, to guide them on their path to specialization in clinical neuropsychology.

—**Scott A. Sperling, PsyD, ABPP-CN,** Center for Neurological Restoration, Neurological Institute, Cleveland Clinic, Cleveland, OH

An essential resource for aspiring neuropsychologists, this workbook provides a clear, step-by-step guide to becoming a neuropsychologist from early preparation in high school and undergraduate to applying to graduate programs, internships, and fellowships, to obtaining licensure and professional board certification. Packed with practical tips, strategies, and worksheets, it helps readers plan, organize, and track their progress with ease. Like having a personal advisor or coach by your side, this book simplifies a complex journey into an achievable roadmap for success in neuropsychology.

—**David S. Sabsevitz, PhD, ABPP,** Associate Professor, Department of Psychiatry & Psychology, Joint Appointment in Neurosurgery, College of Medicine, Mayo Clinic, Jacksonville, FL

This workbook is an essential companion to the parent volume, *The Neuropsychologist's Roadmap: A Training and Career Guide*. It builds on the book as the authors now give you practical and direct intel you need to move through the many stages of the professional neuropsychologist's journey. The authors share important considerations for pursuing each step, but they also share the rationale of why and how their tips lead to success. This workbook importantly evens the playing field in a competitive profession and allows everyone access to personalized specialty-specific professional coaching!

—**Beth K. Rush, PhD, ABPP,** Department of Psychiatry & Psychology, Mayo Clinic, Jacksonville, FL

The Neuropsychologist's Workbook fills a critical gap by highlighting examples of the multiple steps involved in becoming a clinical neuropsychologist. Covering key topics like preparing graduate school applications, navigating internships and postdoctoral fellowships, obtaining licensure, and achieving board certification, it concludes with practical advice on securing a first position in neuropsychology. These blueprints enable aspiring neuropsychologists to avoid missteps, stay on track, and establish the necessary foundation for a fulfilling neuropsychology career in a variety of professional settings.

—**David W. Loring, PhD, ABPP-CN,** Professor, Departments of Neurology and Pediatrics, and Neuropsychology Program Director (Neurology), Emory University School of Medicine, Atlanta, GA

The
Neuropsychologist's
Workbook

*A Hands-On Roadmap to Training
and Developing Your Career*

Cady Block and Sabrina Hickle

AMERICAN PSYCHOLOGICAL ASSOCIATION

Published by
American Psychological Association
750 First Street, NE
Washington, DC 20002
https://www.apa.org

Order Department
https://www.apa.org/pubs/books
order@apa.org

Typeset in Meridien and Ortodoxa by Circle Graphics, Inc., Reisterstown, MD

Printer: Gasch Printing, Odenton, MD
Cover Designer: Gwen J. Grafft, Minneapolis, MN

Library of Congress Cataloging-in-Publication Data

Names: Block, Cady, author. | Hickle, Sabrina, author.
Title: The neuropsychologist's workbook : a hands-on roadmap to training
   and developing your career / by Cady Block and Sabrina Hickle.
Description: Washington, DC : American Psychological Association, [2025] |
   Includes bibliographical references and index.
Identifiers: LCCN 2024037775 (print) | LCCN 2024037776 (ebook) | ISBN
   9781433840128 (paperback) | ISBN 9781433840135 (ebook)
Subjects: MESH: Neuropsychology | Vocational Guidance | Education, Graduate
   | Credentialing
Classification: LCC RC336 (print) | LCC RC336 (ebook) | NLM WL 103.5 |
   DDC 616.80078--dc23/eng/20241230
LC record available at https://lccn.loc.gov/2024037775
LC ebook record available at https://lccn.loc.gov/2024037776

https://doi.org/10.1037/0000448-000

Printed in the United States of America

10 9 8 7 6 5 4 3 2 1

CONTENTS

ACKNOWLEDGMENTS

SABRINA HICKLE

Writing a book is a journey that involves the support, guidance, and encouragement of many people. I am deeply grateful to everyone who has been a part of this process. First, I would like to thank my personal mentors, who have supported me through my training and career. In particular, I'd like to thank Tricia King, who introduced me to Cady during happy hour and suggested that we collaborate on a book. Also, a huge thank you to Suzanne Penna, who has been such an integral part of my neuropsychology journey. Thank you for picking up my slack with good humor when I holed myself in my office to write.

To my colleagues, friends, and trainees, especially Lise De Wit, Becca Huber, Kayci Vickers, Jess Saurman, and Anny Reyes: Thank you for sharing your perspectives, comments, insightful answers to my questions, and for providing feedback and beta testing on our survey.

To my coauthor, Cady Block, who I will forever consider my writing twin. Thank you for your meticulous attention to detail, your feedback, resources, encouragement, and patience during those weeks when life just constantly seemed to get in the way of writing. Our collaboration has been an incredible experience, and I am thrilled that we had the opportunity to work on this together.

And finally, to my loved ones. Wesley, my husband, to whom I dedicate this book. Your support, love, and encouragement made this possible. And to my parents, who sacrificed so much to let me follow my passions and dreams—thank you.

CADY BLOCK

This workbook truly adds something unique to the field of neuropsychology: a portable means by which expert-level information and advice are translated into practical, hands-on activities to help our current and future trainees discover new insights, realize personal values, articulate goals, and facilitate progress along the training journey. It is my hope that trainees find this to be an essential tool and valuable companion to its parent text, *The Neuropsychologist's Roadmap: A Training and Career Guide* (Block, 2021).

The opportunity to add this workbook to *The Neuropsychologist's Roadmap: A Training and Career Guide* was both an honor and a privilege. I am grateful to the staff at the American Psychological Association (APA) for believing in my vision and for their patience as the writing process unfolded. Many amazing people within APA work hard to bring publications to life, and I would like to express special thanks and gratitude to our acquisitions editor Chris Kelaher, as well as to our development editor Krissy Jones. Thank you both for your support and expertise! We couldn't have reached the finish line without you.

I echo Dr. Hickle's expression of thanks for the beta testers of our survey. We also thank all the clinical supervisors and training directors who took time out of their busy schedules to respond with the feedback, input, experience, advice, and wisdom that infuses the pages of our workbook. You are the people from whom trainees most want to hear, and I am sure they will be as appreciative as we are.

Of course, this workbook wouldn't exist without the indefatigable Dr. Sabrina Hickle. When I first pitched her the idea of this workbook, she didn't hesitate to jump in with both feet. I couldn't have asked for a better coauthor! Her enthusiasm is matched only by her writing and organizational skills, and to this day, I remain in awe of her frontal lobes. Thank you, Sabrina, for your contribution and your friendship. We did it!

And finally, many thanks for the love and support provided by other friends and family. You all have been my emotional rock as *The Neuropsychologist's Roadmap* came to life, and again as this workbook developed. I dedicate this to my mother in particular, who has been my never-ending cheerleader in life. This is for you, Mom.

The
Neuropsychologist's
Workbook

1

On Becoming a Neuropsychologist

This book is designed to be a companion to *The Neuropsychologist's Roadmap: A Training and Career Guide* (Block, 2021). As a workbook, it will serve as a practical and more applied guide to help you move through the various steps in the journey to becoming a neuropsychologist. Throughout this book, you will come across clinical material that has been adequately disguised to protect client identity. If you've picked up this workbook or its companion text, you must be seriously considering a career in neuropsychology. We're glad you found us! Neuropsychology is an exciting, intellectually stimulating, diverse, and rewarding profession. But what exactly is neuropsychology?

DEFINITION OF NEUROPSYCHOLOGY

Neuropsychology is a branch of psychology that involves the study of brain and behavior relationships. It draws from a diverse array of disciplines, including psychology, philosophy, neurology, and neuroscience. It is both a science and practice. It is science in that it involves the experimental study of what happens to the brain when it is injured or ailing and how we can enhance brain health and daily function. Neuropsychology is also concerned with the study of how the healthy brain functions, adapts, and maintains its well-being and how a healthy brain supports cognitive processes, behaviors, and emotions. In this way, it is related to other research professions such as neuroscience. It is also a clinical specialty, involving the care of patients and their

https://doi.org/10.1037/0000448-001
The Neuropsychologist's Workbook: A Hands-On Roadmap to Training and Developing Your Career, by C. Block and S. Hickle

families. In this way, it is related to other health professions, such as neurology, psychiatry, rehabilitative therapies, and counseling.

Neuropsychologists wear a lot of hats. We are diagnosticians, interventionists, scientists/researchers, educators, consultants, and advocates. We work in a variety of settings—university or college departments, medical centers associated with universities or colleges (or what we call an "academic medical center"), private or community hospitals, children's hospitals, rehabilitation hospitals/centers, Veterans Affairs medical centers, and private practice. We also are found in the active duty military, the Department of Defense, government agencies (e.g., the Federal Bureau of Investigation, the National Aeronautics and Space Administration, federal prisons), and in industry consulting firms. Neuropsychologists can also be involved in forensic work—they can work with attorneys, courts, and other legal professionals (in civil and criminal matters) to provide expertise on matters where brain function and behavior are in question. As you can see, this leaves the door open to a lot of different career options once you decide on neuropsychology.

One of the mainstays of neuropsychology as a specialty is the neuropsychological assessment, which assesses a range of domains using a multicomponent approach (see Exhibit 1.1). Assessments are used to answer a variety of questions. Here are just some of the scenarios in which a neuropsychologist may be asked to conduct an assessment and the types of questions that they are asked to answer with their assessment:

- Ms. Shah is a 70-year-old woman who is attending her annual physical exam. Her daughter came to the appointment and voices some concerns about her mother's memory. Specifically, she says that Ms. Shah has gotten lost driving home from church. She's noticed that her mother keeps asking the same questions repeatedly. Ms. Shah is referred for a neuropsychological assessment to determine whether these changes reflect normal aging, or if this could be the onset of a neurodegenerative condition—and if so, which one?

- Mr. Porgie is a 45-year-old man who suffered a stroke a year ago. Before his stroke, he worked as a high-level executive at a large company. Immediately after the stroke, he noticed problems with his attention and memory. Even though he feels he has made huge strides in the past year with his therapies, he isn't quite sure whether he can return to work in his previous role. His speech therapist refers Mr. Porgie for a neuropsychological assessment to help determine whether he is ready to return to work.

- Rosie Posie is going into the third grade. She has a history of seizures, which are fairly well controlled with medication, but she is starting to fall behind in school. In the past few months, she has been having meltdowns every day after school. Her epileptologist refers her to a neuropsychologist to help determine what might be driving her recent changes.

As you can see, assessments are used for a variety of reasons, including but not limited to establishing or confirming a diagnosis, assisting with differential

EXHIBIT 1.1

Neuropsychological Assessment Components and Domains

Assessment Components

- *Clinical interview:* This interview involves meeting with the patient, and maybe also including a friend or family member, to gain background and other historical information to provide context to their cognitive changes and test results. The clinical interview covers recent/current changes in thinking (cognition), emotional well-being or personality, behavior, and ability to perform daily activities. It also covers recent medical circumstances, medical or psychiatric diagnoses in the patient and their family history, medications, brain imaging and other lab results, developmental history, school and work history, and current living situation (among other things).

- *Behavioral observations:* These are recorded observations of any cognitive, behavioral, or emotional concerns that arise during the clinical interview or testing. Is the patient alert or confused? Do they seem depressed and tearful, anxious, or irritable? Do they handle difficult tests well, or do they get frustrated easily? Are there any sensory or physical issues interfering with testing, such as vision problems or hand tremors? And so on.

- *Testing:* The neuropsychologist then conducts testing, although many instead use a trained test technician (a psychometrist), one-on-one with the patient. This entails a whole battery of tests that sample the various domains listed later in the table. Testing can take anywhere from 1 hour to 8 or more hours, although appointment length has trended downward as the field and health care in general have evolved over time.

- *Neuropsychological report:* After testing is done, the neuropsychologist reviews and integrates information and data collected during the interview, testing, and through behavioral observations. They produce a final report that is then provided to the person or agency that requested the assessment. This report contains a summarization of test results with data, explanation of what those results mean, and recommendations to enhance medical care, improve daily functioning, and develop a follow-up plan if needed.

- *Feedback:* After the report is complete, the neuropsychologist typically meets again with the patient and family to review findings and recommendations. This provides an opportunity for the patient and family to ask questions.

Assessment Domains

- Orientation to person, time, place, and circumstance
- Sensory and motor functioning
- Intellectual functioning
- Academic achievement
- Speech and language
- Visuospatial and constructional skills
- Attention and working memory
- Processing speed
- Verbal learning and memory
- Nonverbal/visual learning and memory
- Executive functioning
- Mood and personality
- Behavioral health

diagnosis, providing a baseline for tracking purposes, determining one's ability to perform activities of daily living (e.g., basic tasks such as brushing one's hair up to more complex ones like driving, managing medications, paying bills, and attending medical appointments), determining one's decision-making ability (e.g., for financial or medical decisions), documenting deficits for disability benefits or accommodations to make work or school more manageable, determining candidacy or risk as part of a presurgical workup, and assisting in treatment planning.

Neuropsychologists are also often engaged in treatment. For instance, they conduct psychotherapy to help someone adjust to a new diagnosis or its associated cognitive, emotional, and functional deficits. They also conduct cognitive rehabilitation/remediation treatment, which is a special form of therapy that helps directly address cognitive deficits—by helping someone recover as much as possible or by compensating for what cannot be recovered by utilizing their cognitive strengths and other available tools and technologies.

Neuropsychologists are also involved in research, education, and mentorship. Some examples of research studies in which they may be involved include the following:

- Studying the efficacy of new medications or therapeutic interventions for neurological disorders.

- Using neuroimaging techniques such as functional magnetic resonance imaging to investigate brain function in clinical populations at rest or during specific tasks.

- Tracking individuals over time to understand how neurological conditions progress and how they impact cognition and behavior, as well as which factors increase or decrease risk of progression.

- Investigating the neural basis of cognitive functions such as attention, language, learning, and memory.

- Examining neurological disorders that have a genetic basis and identifying genetic markers associated with these conditions; exploring how the brain develops in infants, children, and adolescents and how genetic and environmental factors influence outcomes

- Investigating the brain's potential to reorganize itself after injury or disease and developing rehabilitation strategies to optimize recovery.

- Exploring how cultural factors influence brain structure, function, behavior, and test performance.

A day in the life of a neuropsychologist can look different based on the setting and what portion of their time is spent on which of these tasks because often, neuropsychologists are involved in several of these activities. Here is what a day might look like across several different neuropsychologists:

- Dr. Vasquez is a neuropsychologist in the psychology department at ABC University. She has several grants that support her work on the neuro-imaging of brain tumors. She trains graduate students in her lab. She teaches two courses in the graduate clinical psychology program. She also supervises several assessment cases in the university training clinic.

- Dr. Smith is a neuropsychologist at XYZ Rehabilitation Center. It is a private facility, but he holds an appointment at a nearby medical school. He performs a combination of cognitive rehabilitation and assessment in persons with brain injury, stroke, and multiple sclerosis. He also does some legal consultations on the side.

- Dr. Azarenka is a clinical neuropsychologist in the neurology department at the School of Medicine. They conduct 8 to 10 assessments per week. They also attend and present at educational events, such as case conferences. They are also involved in training; they conduct supervision every week with their trainees and review their testing and reports. They also collaborate on a research study with other neurologists in the department.

NEUROPSYCHOLOGY AND RELATED PROFESSIONS

You may be asking how a neuropsychologist may differ from other health professions. There are many points of overlap in that they work with individuals with neurological and psychiatric conditions, but there are some crucial differences.

Neuropsychology Versus Neurology

Both neuropsychologists and neurologists serve clinical patients with neurological disorders and diseases. Neurology primarily deals with the medical aspects of neurological disorders, focusing on diagnosis and medical treatment (e.g., medications, surgery). A neuropsychologist focuses on assessing the cognitive, emotional, and behavioral impact of the condition on daily life. When a neuropsychologist is involved in treatment, they use cognitive rehabilitation techniques and behavioral interventions. The pathway to a career in neuropsychology involves a doctoral degree with further specialization in neuropsychology. Neurology involves medical school followed by a residency in neurology. Additional fellowships may be pursued for specialized areas within neurology.

Neuropsychology Versus Psychiatry

Both neuropsychologists and psychiatrists work with patients who have mental health/psychiatric conditions. Psychiatry concentrates on diagnosing and treating mental health conditions through medication management and sometimes various forms of therapy. Similar to neurology, the training pathway involves medical school, followed by a residency in psychiatry.

Neuropsychology Versus Occupational or Speech Therapy

Occupational therapists (OTs) and speech/language pathologists (SLPs) also work with patients who are affected by neurological (and other medical) conditions. An OT's emphasis is on assessing and restoring a person's ability to perform daily activities, enhancing their engagement in self-care, work, and other activities. OTs work directly with their patients to teach techniques, how to use adaptive equipment, and ways to modify the environment to improve their ability to perform their daily activities independently. SLPs specialize in communication and swallowing disorders. They also work directly with their patients, creating treatment plans and using various exercises to improve speech, language, and swallowing abilities. The pathway to be an OT or SLP typically involves master's level training.

Neuropsychology Versus Psychometry

A psychometrist typically works under the supervision of a psychologist. They serve the same patient population. A psychometrist administers and scores assessment measures, but they do not interpret results, make diagnoses, develop treatment plans, or (typically) write reports. The training pathway typically involves a bachelor's or master's degree.

As you can see, there are many points of overlap between these professions. Which profession you pick really depends on your interests, the degree to which you want to be involved in patient care and treatment, and your ability to devote time to a specific training pathway. If you like neuropsychological assessment and working directly with patients but don't want to spend 6 to 8 years training, you may enjoy being a psychometrist. If you like working one-on-one with neurological populations but are not interested in medical school and don't like the idea of conducting neuropsychological assessments, you may enjoy being an OT or SLP. If you love the brain and cognition but are not keen on the idea of clinical work, you may enjoy being a neuroscientist or experimental psychologist.

THE JOURNEY TO BECOMING A NEUROPSYCHOLOGIST

Becoming a neuropsychologist requires dedication, extensive education, and practical training. The typical pathway to becoming a neuropsychologist involves an undergraduate degree (e.g., bachelor's degree in psychology, neuroscience, or a related field) focusing on coursework in neuroscience, research methods, and psychology. At least in the United States, the next step is a doctoral graduate program—ideally one that has specialized coursework in neuropsychology (i.e., assessment, neuroanatomy) and has neuropsychologists that can serve as supervisors and mentors, as well as neuropsychology practica (a supervised training experience that offers hands-on opportunities to learn neuropsychological knowledge and skills). The final year of graduate training is internship, which involves 1 year of full-time work at a new institution. Neuropsychologists are also expected to complete 2 years of postdoctoral training for further specialization, which is necessary for board certification.

Our workbook is organized by each step of the training journey to becoming a neuropsychologist, so we have a chapter each dedicated to early preparation (i.e., high school and undergrad), graduate school, internship, and postdoctoral fellowship. We also cover topics in the early career phase and have a chapter each on licensure, board certification, and the first job. Within each of these chapters, we include information, advice, and activities designed to help you assess and improve your readiness to apply to the next step, locate and apply to programs/positions, practice interview skills, and identify any potential roadblocks. We wanted to ensure that our book was timely, relevant, and data driven. So before writing this workbook, we created a survey and sent it out to actual directors/codirectors and supervisors within neuropsychology training programs who are involved in the review and selection of applicants for graduate school, internship, and postdoctoral fellowship or in the review and selection of neuropsychology job candidates to ensure that the advice provided in this book is up-to-date, accurate, and timely. Fifty-seven neuropsychologists[1] responded, and we've infused their advice into each of our chapters. As a nice complement to the broad overview provided in *The Neuropsychologist's Roadmap*, you will find many visual aids, thought exercises, worksheets, and checklists that you can use to aid you on your journey to becoming a neuropsychologist. To get the most out of this workbook, we recommend that you actively engage with the materials. For our thought exercises and brainstorming activities, take the time to review the prompts and write down what you are thinking. Use our sample materials as a starting point, but make sure to adapt them so they are personalized for your needs and setting. Feel free to make copies of worksheets, tables, and checklists. These are designed to help you organize everything effectively, and they will help you be systematic as you check off items to make sure you don't miss an important step. And between this workbook and the main text, you will be well-prepared to conquer each step of that journey!

---

[1]If you would like group-level data on respondent demographics and information about the training programs, please email the authors (Block.cady@mayo.edu or s.diana.na@gmail.com).

2

Early Preparation

High School and Undergraduate

 Before working through activities on this topic, be sure to read through Chapter 1 of this workbook, which details the neuropsychology educational and training pathway.

This chapter is designed for the earliest of us: people in high school, college, or immediately after college who think they may be interested in neuropsychology. If you are reading this book, you are likely seriously considering this as a career path. How can you be sure that this is the right career? Here, we provide an overview of the educational and training pathway and what sort of experiences make you competitive for graduate school down the line.

THE NEUROPSYCHOLOGY EDUCATIONAL AND TRAINING PATHWAY

In thinking about whether neuropsychology is the right career for you, you need to know what sort of commitment you're making. Training to be a neuropsychologist is a huge personal and financial commitment. Graduate school, which is a requirement on your road to becoming a neuropsychologist, is an exercise in delayed gratification—never mind additional steps along the way such as internship, postdoctoral fellowship, licensure, and board certification. In many ways, the journey is akin to those in medical school. In fact, the training model for doctoral programs in clinical psychology (or other related applied psychology fields such as counseling or community psychology) was structured similarly. As you can see in Figure 2.1, both include a foundational step with subsequent training experiences and tests/licensure processes—all leading to the highest designation of competence in the field, board certification.

https://doi.org/10.1037/0000448-002
The Neuropsychologist's Workbook: A Hands-On Roadmap to Training and Developing Your Career, by C. Block and S. Hickle

FIGURE 2.1. Medical School Versus Graduate Psychology Educational and Training Pathway

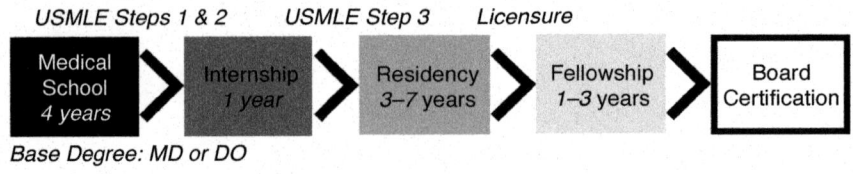

USMLE Steps 1 & 2 · USMLE Step 3 · Licensure

Medical School 4 years › Internship *1 year* › Residency *3–7 years* › Fellowship *1–3 years* › Board Certification

Base Degree: MD or DO

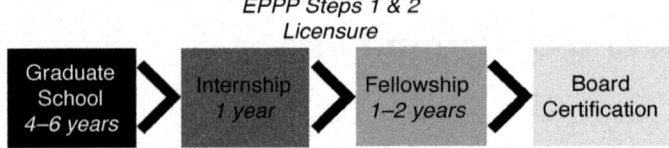

EPPP Steps 1 & 2
Licensure

Graduate School 4–6 years › Internship *1 year* › Fellowship *1–2 years* › Board Certification

Base Degree: PhD or PsyD (clinical, counseling, or community psychology)

Note. EPPP = Examination for Professional Practice in Psychology; USMLE = U.S. Medical Licensing Examination.

Mapping out the psychology trajectory in more detail (see Figure 2.2), we can see that each of these steps involves a range of requisite educational coursework and didactics, research training experiences, and clinical training experiences. All in all, you can expect a roughly 7- to 9-year educational/training commitment, not including additional time spent completing the board certification process. It might seem overwhelming at first, but the right mindset with a dose of persistence, mentorship, and resources does make it more manageable.

A few caveats: Please refer to "The Neuropsychology Educational and Training Pathway" section in Chapter 3 of this workbook for some specific considerations about the type of doctoral program you will attend because this does make a difference for your ultimate career. It bears mentioning that there is no neuropsychology doctoral degree to be obtained; rather, the doctoral degree is typically in a broader applied psychology specialty such as clinical psychology, counseling psychology, community psychology, and others (you can think about it like medical school, where your degree is "medical doctor/MD" and then you complete residency and fellowship to specialize in an area such as cardiology or neurology). The same goes for neuropsychology, where you may obtain some experience along the way but ultimately specialize in your postdoctoral fellowship years. It is possible to become a neuropsychologist even after all those educational/training pathway steps are complete. For people who went a different path but want to switch to neuropsychology, you can complete what is called a *respecialization program* (see https://www.apa.org/ed/graduate/respecialization).

Next, while postdoctoral fellowships across psychology specialties can range anywhere from 1 to 2 years, in neuropsychology, the expectation is that you will complete a 2-year fellowship. And finally, to practice psychology professionally

FIGURE 2.2. Graduate Applied Psychology Educational and Training Pathway

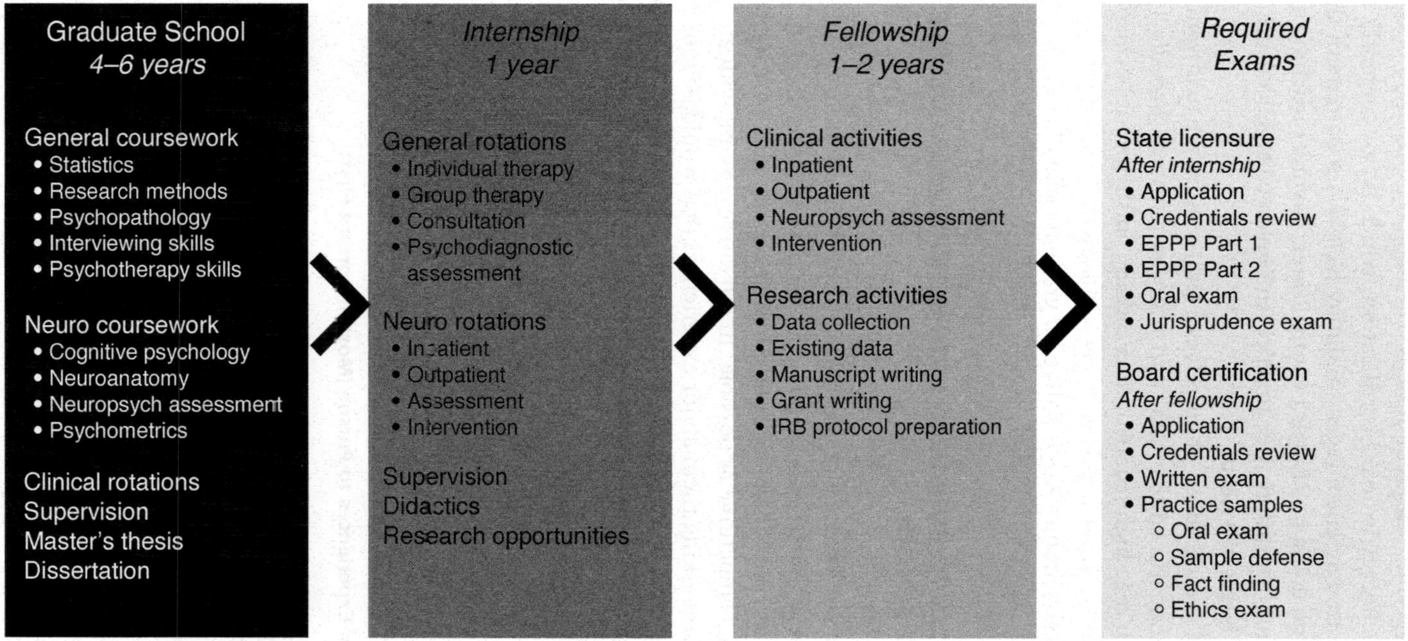

Graduate School
4–6 years

General coursework
- Statistics
- Research methods
- Psychopathology
- Interviewing skills
- Psychotherapy skills

Neuro coursework
- Cognitive psychology
- Neuroanatomy
- Neuropsych assessment
- Psychometrics

Clinical rotations
Supervision
Master's thesis
Dissertation

Internship
1 year

General rotations
- Individual therapy
- Group therapy
- Consultation
- Psychodiagnostic assessment

Neuro rotations
- Inpatient
- Outpatient
- Assessment
- Intervention

Supervision
Didactics
Research opportunities

Fellowship
1–2 years

Clinical activities
- Inpatient
- Outpatient
- Neuropsych assessment
- Intervention

Research activities
- Data collection
- Existing data
- Manuscript writing
- Grant writing
- IRB protocol preparation

Required Exams

State licensure
After internship
- Application
- Credentials review
- EPPP Part 1
- EPPP Part 2
- Oral exam
- Jurisprudence exam

Board certification
After fellowship
- Application
- Credentials review
- Written exam
- Practice samples
  - Oral exam
  - Sample defense
  - Fact finding
  - Ethics exam

Base Degree: PhD or PsyD (clinical, counseling, or community psychology)

Note. EPPP = Examination for Professional Practice in Psychology; IRB = institutional review board.

you must be licensed. This requires completion of a national examination called the Examination for Professional Practice in Psychology as well as some additional state-specific examination steps. The highest designation of competency in neuropsychology is board certification, which is not currently a requirement but is strongly encouraged (and may well be a requirement someday so best to plan on doing it). If your eventual career involves teaching or research in an academic institution, then practice isn't involved and licensure and board certification is less of a need.

But we're getting ahead of ourselves a bit. For now, we just want you to be aware of what the educational and training pathway broadly looks like. Whether you're in high school or have already finished your bachelor's degree, there are myriad ways to engage in psychology to learn more about the field and make yourself more competitive for graduate school.

EXPERIENCES TO PURSUE IN HIGH SCHOOL AND COLLEGE BEFORE GRADUATE SCHOOL

Let's assume you've decided neuropsychology is the right career path for you. It's good you're thinking about this early because getting into graduate school is tough, and you will need to be proactive in seeking out experiences to make you as competitive as possible. In our survey, 57 individuals responded to the question asking them about experiences that would be most important for high schoolers, undergraduates, and postbaccalaureates to pursue if they are interested in a career in neuropsychology. We've summarized their results in Exhibit 2.1.

EXHIBIT 2.1

Survey Results: Ranked Graduate School Application Factors

Top 3 Ranked Experiences to Pursue (Most Important First)

1. Neuropsychology research experiences (e.g., neuropsychology research lab assistant)
2. Neuropsychology clinical experiences (e.g., shadowing a neuropsychologist)
3. Having a degree major in psychology or neuroscience

Bottom Ranked Factors (Least Important First)

1. Taking other related college courses (e.g., advanced statistics, computer programming, biology)
2. Attending a neuropsychology, neuroscience, or psychology conference
3. Other nonneuropsychology clinical experiences (e.g., crisis counseling, youth advocacy, therapy)
4. Other nonneuropsychology research experiences (e.g., general psychological or neuroscience)

Research Experiences

As you can see, gaining relevant neuropsychology research experience was deemed important: 85% of people filling out our survey ranked it as one of their top three recommendations. What does "relevant" neuropsychological research mean? This typically means research in which you are investigating brain–behavior relationships and exploring cognitive functions (i.e., memory, attention, perception).

Of course, you want to demonstrate that you have experience in the day-to-day aspects of helping run a research study—these are things such as recruiting participants, getting informed consents, collecting data, and entering data into a database. You also want to demonstrate that you have some familiarity with the steps of the scientific process—of reviewing and synthesizing pre-existing scientific literature, coming up with a research question, analyzing data by using the appropriate statistical tests, and communicating your results. Even if you do not intend to perform scientific research as part of your career, a core competency for all doctoral programs is that you are able to consume and interpret scientific research. The best and easiest way for you to demonstrate that you have this important skill is with a *research product*, such as a poster, presentation, or paper. This is why 83% of our survey participants indicated that a competitive applicant to their program had at least one publication, oral presentation, or poster.

How do you go about gaining research experience? We recommend that you look up research studies being conducted around you. A good first place to look is at an academic institution or university. Look at the website for faculty members in the psychology or neuroscience departments. Their websites usually have pages devoted to active research studies. If you do not see any neuropsychology-specific labs, that's okay. You can look for labs that give you experience with neuropsychological clinical populations (patients with conditions that affect the brain or have known effects on cognition, such as stroke and traumatic brain injury; adults with Alzheimer's disease; children with learning disabilities); study cognitive domains, such as attention, memory, executive functioning; or give you experience in more advanced statistical methods (e.g., structural equation modeling) or techniques (e.g., neuroimaging or genomics). Another option would be to look outside of your institution. Are there hospitals near you, such as a Veterans Affairs (VA) hospital or an academic medical center? Look through the website to see if there are any neuropsychologists (typically in the psychiatry or neurology department) involved in research. Even if their website does not mention research studies, it is worth reaching out to individuals to ask if they are actively involved in research and may need a research assistant. Even if they say no, they could put you in touch with someone else who is looking for one.

Email that person introducing yourself and expressing your interest in their research. Ask if they are taking on any research assistants. If yes, interview and ask if there might be opportunities for you to work on a poster or manuscript. Do not be surprised if you are told that you are expected to do this outside of your regular lab hours. Working on a poster or manuscript is considered a bonus opportunity in many labs because they often require additional mentorship. If they say no, consider whether there may be other labs that could provide more relevant research experience. If there truly are no realistic ways for you to get research experience in neuropsychology, know that any research experience in a different field of psychology, sociology, or a related field is better than none.

When you join a research lab, the research mentor will likely be an important letter writer for your application, so this means that you need to be professional and conscientious. Show up on time, and complete the tasks required of you. Here are some things we would recommend you do to maximize your experiences in the lab. First, keep track of the types of tasks you do in the lab because you'll want to put that information on your resumé. Second, if you have mastered a particular task, ask for other responsibilities so you can gain proficiency in other areas of research. Third, express your interest in working on a research poster or manuscript early and often! Sometimes the research lab is in the data collecting phase when you join, and they may not have any data available for you to analyze at that time. But by (gently—don't go overboard!) reminding your mentors that you are interested, they will think of you and ideally will loop you in when they are ready to publish. You can use the checklist provided in Exhibit 2.2 to help you keep track of the types of research tasks you have mastered and to help guide you as to which types of tasks you would want to get experience and mastery in next.

There are research opportunities at every level (see Table 2.1) although, admittedly, this can be more challenging at the high school than the college level. If you are in high school, we suggest looking up your state's psychological association and asking them what opportunities exist for you locally. Some universities (such as the University of Chicago, Rice University, and Georgia State University) offer summer psychology or neuroscience courses

---

EXHIBIT 2.2

Checklist of Research Competencies

☐   Recruiting participants (e.g., creating flyers/ads; calling people to gauge interest)

☐   Getting informed consent

☐   Writing up the IRB application

☐   Running an experiment

☐   Collecting data

☐   Entering data into a database

☐   Conducting a literature review

☐   Analyzing data

☐   Creating a poster

☐   Writing a manuscript or writing sections of a manuscript

Note. IRB = institutional review board—an internal board at your institution that reviews research studies to ensure that they are feasible and ethically sound.

TABLE 2.1. Opportunities for High Schoolers, Undergraduates, and Postbaccalaureates

Level	Opportunities
High school	• State Psychological Associations: https://www.apa.org/about/apa/organizations/associations • Society for Neuroscience: https://www.sfn.org/meetings/neuroscience-2022/registration/registration-categories • NIH Summer Internship Program: https://www.training.nih.gov/research-training/hs/hs-sip/histep • Barrow Summer Internship: https://www.barrowneuro.org/for-physicians-researchers/research/training-programs/high-school-research-program • sci-MI Neuroscience Summer Program: https://sci-mi.github.io/nmp.html • Pathways To Science list: https://www.pathwaystoscience.org/Discipline.aspx?sort=SOC-PsychBehavSci_Psychology%20*%20Behavioral%20Sciences
Undergraduate	• State Psychological Associations: https://www.apa.org/about/apa/organizations/associations • Psi Chi: https://www.psichi.org • Harvard Multicultural Alzheimer's Prevention Program: https://mapp.mgh.harvard.edu/training • Rutgers University RISE Program: https://www.rise.rutgers.edu • sci-MI Neuroscience Summer Program: https://sci-mi.github.io/nmp.html • American Psychological Association list: https://www.apa.org/education-career/undergrad/research-opportunities • Pathways To Science list: https://www.pathwaystoscience.org/Discipline.aspx?sort=SOC-PsychBehavSci_Psychology%20*%20Behavioral%20Sciences
Postbaccalaureate	• NIH Postbac Program: https://www.training.nih.gov/research-training/pb/pb • MINDS Program: https://med.umn.edu/neuroscience/diversity-inclusion/training-career-research • PREP Program list: https://www.nigms.nih.gov/maps/Pages/Post-Baccalaureate-Research-Education-Program-Institutions.aspx

Note. NIH = National Institutes of Health.

for high school students. Less commonly, hospitals offer supervised research opportunities, such as the one offered through the Barrow Clinic in Arizona. The National Institutes of Health sponsors a summer internship program in biomedical research, open to high school juniors or seniors aged 17 or older; this program is an opportunity to be paid to learn about scientific research. Attending research conferences is also not out of the realm of possibility: the Society for Neuroscience allows chaperoned high schoolers to attend their annual meeting!

At the undergraduate level, state psychological associations and the Society for Neuroscience conference are also available. But now, other opportunities start to present themselves. There is of course the option of volunteering to be a research assistant in the lab of one of the faculty at your university or college.

You can also now become involved in Psi Chi, the national honor society for psychology. There are also training programs and internships available, such as the ones listed by the American Psychological Association or Pathways to Science. Some of these are dedicated to individuals from historically underrepresented backgrounds, such as the Harvard Multicultural Alzheimer's Prevention Program (MAPP) or the RISE program through Rutgers University.

For those who are post-baccalaureate, the National Institutes of Health has a postbaccalaureate program that funds 1 to 2 years of mentored research. The University of Minnesota sponsors the Inclusive Neuroscience Development Scholars (MINDS) program, which provides financial support for college graduates to conduct 2 years of research in a neuroscience laboratory at the University of Minnesota before pursuing a PhD in neuroscience or related field. For historically underrepresented people, the National Institutes of Health PREP Program funds gap-year experiences with support in research and mentoring. There are others, but these are good places to begin your search.

Clinical Experiences

The next important experience to get in this stage is neuropsychology clinical experience, such as shadowing a neuropsychologist. This will help you get a clearer sense of the day-to-day experience for a neuropsychologist and whether this is something that you can see yourself doing long term. These experiences will not only help you figure out whether this is the correct career path for you, but they will help demonstrate to the people reviewing your application to graduate school that you are serious about neuropsychology. Here is a step-by-step guide for how to gain valuable shadowing experience.

1. **Research and reach out:** First, identify a list of potential neuropsychologists. There are several places to look; try the websites of local academic, research, and VA hospitals; mental health clinics; and universities. You may have to look within departments like neurology or psychiatry. You can also try searching professors or advisors within psychology or neuroscience departments in a university. Once you have a list, reach out to them via email. Be concise and professional in your communication. Explain your interest in neuropsychology and your desire to shadow to gain insight into the field. Be prepared for the possibility of multiple attempts or rejections before securing an opportunity. We've provided a sample email that you can use (Exhibit 2.3). You can tailor the email to reflect your genuine interest and respect for their work, which will increase your chances of a positive response.

2. **Prepare professionally:** Dress professionally; in a health care setting, it's typically business casual with closed-toe shoes. Always be on time.

3. **Be proactive:** Ask lots and lots of questions. This is your opportunity to learn. Prepare questions beforehand and ask them at appropriate moments. Pay attention to the interactions between the neuropsychologist and patients. Note their communication style, methods, and techniques. Bring a notebook

EXHIBIT 2.3

Shadowing Request Email Template

[Your Name] Subject: Request to Shadow a Neuropsychologist

Dear Dr. [Last Name]:

I hope this message finds you well. My name is [Your Name], and I am currently a [high school/college] student at [Your School/University]. I am in the process of exploring careers in health care and am particularly interested in the field of neuropsychology. I am seeking out opportunities to shadow and gain firsthand insight into the day-to-day responsibilities of a neuropsychologist in a clinical setting. If you are willing and your clinic allows students to shadow, I would appreciate any opportunity to observe your work, even for a brief period.

Thank you very much for considering my request. Please let me know if there's any further information you require from me.

Warm regards,

[Your Full Name]

[Your Contact Information]

[Your School/University, if applicable]

and ask if you are allowed to take notes. Jot down key observations, interesting cases, or methodologies (if permitted).

4. **Follow-up and express gratitude:** After shadowing, send an email expressing gratitude for the opportunity. It leaves a positive impression. If the neuropsychologist tells you that you can continue to stay in touch, stay connected for advice or future opportunities. They may be able to open the door for other opportunities, like additional shadowing or research projects.

We also asked the neuropsychologists who took our survey what you should do if you don't have easy access to these types of experiences. Several people continued to emphasize how crucial it is to have research and clinical experience in neuropsychology and suggested taking extra time and relocating so you can get these experiences. It is not uncommon for people to take several years after undergrad to get the experiences needed to be competitive for graduate school. One person wrote, "Seek out someone to do research with—that is the most important thing, and it is never too late to do so, even if you are no longer in a degree program. I know it is difficult to volunteer and not be paid but even if you can do that for a few hours a week, and end up on conference abstracts and papers, it will be time well spent." Another wrote, "Be creative in how you may be able to access some of these experiences. Although time can be a limitation . . . research experiences may be accessible remotely or in-person during specific times (e.g., I've had students at smaller schools with less research opportunities do research in my lab in the summer if they are from this area and move back home for the summer)."

Others emphasized the importance of one-on-one mentorship. A neuropsychology mentor can serve as a source of knowledge about the training journey and career path, offer support and provide advice, share resources, and help you make connections with the neuropsychology community. There are several ways to go about securing a mentor. One way to do this is to reach out to faculty members at your psychology program whose work seems interesting to you. If you have a chance, ask them about their experience in graduate school, their current work, and any advice they might have. This can often lead to valuable shadowing or research opportunities. Another way to secure a neuropsychology mentor is to check out New2Neuropsychology (N2N, https://new2neuropsych.org), an organization whose objective is to support students in successful matriculation through neuropsychology training programs by providing easy access to practical resources about neuropsychology training, connections to neuropsychologists from underrepresented backgrounds, and warm hand-offs to mentorship and networking opportunities. They have a section on their website devoted to helping students find mentors in neuropsychology, including helpful links to several neuropsychology mentorship programs that are offered by professional organizations. If this feels intimidating and you don't know which mentorship program to pick, you can meet with a student liaison through N2N who can help you determine which mentorship program would be the right fit and help connect you to other resources and opportunities to pursue education and training in neuropsychology.

We also want to highlight something in Exhibit 2.1: There were some experiences that were not selected as the top three most important to pursue. Taking other related college courses (e.g., advanced statistics, computer programming, biology); attending a neuropsychology, neuroscience, or psychology conference; and other nonneuropsychology clinical or research experiences were not rated as the top three most important experiences to pursue. We aren't saying that these experiences are unimportant, worthless, or undesired. In fact, some neuropsychologists could argue that having these additional experiences could help set you apart from your peers when you are applying to graduate programs. But we provide these numbers to help inform you as to which experiences are broadly considered the most important by neuropsychologists so that you can prioritize accordingly. If you've completed all these experiences and realized that perhaps this is not the right career for you, don't be discouraged. You've still gained valuable experience and learned some new skills. Reflect on what you specifically did like, and what you didn't like when you were doing research or shadowing a neuropsychologist. Explore these with your mentor or career counselor—they may help guide you toward exploring a different career option. Trust us, it's better to know at this stage—before you've gone through the application process, possibly taken on student loans, and moved to a different city—that this is not the right career path for you.

PREPARING YOURSELF TO BE COMPETITIVE

Once you have decided that this is the career path you want to pursue, make sure you have a good understanding now on how to be a competitive applicant for graduate school. We recommend that you read *The Neuropsychologist's Roadmap* (Block, 2021; especially the chapters pertaining to preparing for graduate school and the chapters related to foundational competencies in neuropsychology), as well as the next chapter in this workbook. We provide some benchmarks that are typical for a competitive applicant in neuropsychology (e.g., number of posters and publications), as well as the types of experiences that people are looking for when they review applications for graduate school. You can use these numbers as your goals and hatch a plan and timeline to ensure that you use your time effectively now to focus your efforts for the following year(s). This will keep you from scrambling in the months before you apply for graduate school, realizing that it is too late to get the kinds of experiences you need to be competitive. Here are some specific tips:

- **Ensure the right preparatory coursework:** While an undergraduate degree in psychology is not necessarily required, graduate programs still like to see specific foundational psychology courses. These most often include some combination of abnormal psychology or psychopathology, statistics, research design, and biopsychology.

- **Seek out the neuro:** If you want to be a competitive applicant, you want to show that you have neuropsychology-specific experiences. Aim for at least one poster presentation at a conference in the realm of neuropsychology, neuroscience, or neurology. It's even better if you have a publication. This isn't strictly necessary or expected—but if you can get one first author publication, this will really help set you apart from other applicants. At minimum, get some experience shadowing a neuropsychologist. If you want to stand out, try to pursue research or clinical experiences where you will learn how to administer and score neuropsychological tests.

- **Follow the timeline:** Use Table 1.2 in *The Neuropsychologist's Roadmap* for a detailed timeline before applying to graduate school. It recommends starting in the sophomore year of undergrad to make sure you have the recommended clinical and research experiences if you want to be able to start graduate school right after completing your undergraduate degree. But don't panic if you are finding this information much later than sophomore year or undergrad. It's common for people to take some time between undergrad and grad school to gain relevant research and clinical experience.

- **Utilize the resources available at your institution:** You may have a career center that can help you create and provide feedback on your progress, your curriculum vitae (it's like an academic resume), cover letters, and essays. Joining Psi Chi, the International Honor Society in Psychology, may be another option available for resources. Through Psi Chi, you could access psychology mentors, gain leadership and community service experiences, and gain resources to aid in academic and professional development. You may also be able to get financial help—for instance, scholarships and grants to support your travel to a conference. Your institution could also host panels, Q&A sessions, seminars, or other educational opportunities for you to learn more about graduate school, careers in psychology, and applications.

- **Do everything in your power to establish a mentor in neuropsychology:** Other individuals could provide good pointers on how to craft our curriculum vitae and cover letters, but a neuropsychology mentor will be the one providing the most pertinent advice and guidance. A good mentor will be able to have specific discussions about what your career in neuropsychology might look like, help you develop an action plan for how to reach your short- and long-term goals, provide feedback on your progress, brainstorm ways to manage any roadblocks, and help you network. We cannot stress enough how important it is to have a mentor!

- **Be observant:** As you start having research and clinical experiences, take stock of what you enjoy. You don't have to pick one (research or clinical career); many are engaged in both. Many use actual clinical data as the basis for their research; others collect data as part of an original study. You can work in a research lab and run a private practice on the side. However, you do have to emphasize one over the other. It is rare to find a 50% clinical/50% research position. Start thinking about your potential interests and what sorts of activities you want to be doing in your career. That way, you can identify what your training needs are when applying to programs. As an example, if you find that you are fired up about research and want a research-based career in an academic institution, you want to search for programs that have more of a research emphasis and will teach you the skills that you need to be successful in that career (e.g., grant-writing skills). It's harder to pick up grant-writing skills and experience as you get further into your training and career. Early identification of your interests will help you be more intentional in selecting the training programs you need to be successful and fulfilled in your career goals.

3

Applying and Getting Into Graduate School

 Before working through activities on this topic, be sure to read through Chapter 1 of *The Neuropsychologist's Roadmap*. We also advise that you skim Chapters 1 and 2 of this workbook, which touch on the educational/training pathway.

This chapter is all about graduate school (or grad school for short). Getting into grad school is tough—in some instances tougher than medical school. We use the qualifying word "some" here because acceptance rates at clinical psychology programs vary widely by program type. In this chapter, we have provided some practical advice for your application and success in grad school that is infused with feedback from 20 training directors/codirectors and supervisors who filled out our survey and responded to items related to grad school. We present data throughout the chapter to help you better understand what these individuals are looking for in grad school applicants.

THE NEUROPSYCHOLOGY EDUCATIONAL AND TRAINING PATHWAY

As you've read in Chapter 1 of *The Neuropsychologist's Roadmap* (Block, 2021) and Chapters 1 and 2 of this workbook, there is an educational/training pathway that one must follow to become a neuropsychologist. You understand that the first step of this pathway is graduate school, and the traditional path is to enter a doctoral program after you complete your undergraduate degree. Some people do it this way. If you're aiming for this, there are a few important pieces of information to know as you seek to apply to doctoral programs.

First, you'll select the main type of doctoral programs, of which there are two: PhD and PsyD (see Tip 3 in Chapter 1 of *The Neuropsychologist's Roadmap* [pp. 16–17] for more information on the PhD/PsyD distinction). Next, you'll

https://doi.org/10.1037/0000448-003
The Neuropsychologist's Workbook: A Hands-On Roadmap to Training and Developing Your Career, by C. Block and S. Hickle

need to decide on program focus and model. The majority of doctoral psychology programs are in *clinical psychology*, but you will see during your research that there are other program types including *counseling psychology*, *community psychology*, *clinical health psychology*, and *medical–clinical psychology*. We've seen successful neuropsychologists emerge from all of these, so in our opinion, this matters less than whether the program affords you access to the type of specialized coursework (e.g., introduction to neuropsychology, neuropsychological assessment, neuroanatomy, behavioral neuroscience) and training opportunities (clinical and/or research) that you seek. The program model does matter quite a bit, however, because this impacts the emphasis of the program. Models include *scientist–practitioner*, *practitioner–scholar*, and *clinician–scientist*; see pages 172 and 173 (Chapter 9) in *The Neuropsychologist's Roadmap* for more information about the distinction between these.

In terms of suggested resources, we find *The Insider's Guide to Graduate Programs in Clinical and Counseling Psychology* (2022) by John C. Norcross and Michael A. Seyette to be an especially helpful book because it includes a detailed index of doctoral programs and their training model, specific characteristics, opportunities, and so on. This is a broad book, however, and if you want to examine doctoral programs offering education and training in neuropsychology, then we encourage you to check out the free online directory sponsored by the Society for Clinical Neuropsychology (https://scn40.org/training-directory). If you're pursuing neuropsychology specifically, it's good to know about the Houston Conference Guidelines (https://uh.edu/hns/hc.html). This is a document that is the product of a consensus effort by leading neuropsychology organizations and details the knowledge and skills necessary for becoming a neuropsychologist. Between this and the American Psychological Association (APA) Commission for the Recognition of Specialties and Subspecialties in Professional Psychology's (CRSSPP) Taxonomy for Education and Training in Clinical Neuropsychology (for more information, see Sperling et al., 2017), you'll find information here that will be helpful when you're trying to determine whether a program's coursework, clinical opportunities, and research training best serve your ultimate career goal.

ALTERNATE PATHS TO GRADUATE SCHOOL

Not everyone goes straight from an undergraduate to a doctoral program, however. If you learned about neuropsychology later and the college timeline on page 13 of *The Neuropsychologist's Roadmap* doesn't apply to you, don't worry—you haven't missed the boat! It's common for people to take several "gap years" after undergrad before applying to graduate school. Many people work as a research assistant or a psychometrist to clinical patients under the supervision of a neuropsychologist. These options provide a good foundational experience that will make you more competitive for graduate school, especially if this work gives you experience with neuropsychology specifically. Working has the advantage of allowing you to save some money to make your time in graduate school a little bit more comfortable and potentially help you avoid taking out loans.

Some people opt for a terminal master's program in clinical psychology, which is also a viable option to help you get some coursework, clinical, and research experiences. We'd encourage you to weigh the pros and cons of this approach and do your due diligence before applying. If your goal for your master's program is to get the types of experiences that will help you be more competitive for a PhD or PsyD program, you will want to ensure that the master's program will provide relevant experiences. We would hate for you to enroll in a master's program, move, and spend money on the program, only to realize that the program does not provide any of the experiences that we talked about in this chapter to help you be competitive. Review the sections in this book regarding experiences you should pursue before graduate school, as well as the sections on how to become a competitive applicant to determine whether the master's program will check any of these boxes. If it's unclear from the program materials whether the master's program will help you with these experiences, make sure to ask. We will also caution you not to rely on the assumption that having a master's degree will let you skip the coursework and will reduce the amount of time that you spend in the doctorate program. It is not uncommon for people who have completed a master's degree to later encounter difficulty transferring course credits from their master's program to their doctoral program.

One final note about master's programs: There is a persisting myth that graduate programs do not favor people who are currently enrolled in (or have already completed) a master's degree before enrolling in a doctoral program. We asked neuropsychologists in our survey how they viewed applicants with a master's degree when considering them for their graduate program. Fifty-five percent of our survey respondents said that the master's program did not matter how they viewed the applicant, whereas 45 percent indicated that they would view the applicant positively. Nobody responded that they would view the applicant negatively. We hope this helps you make a more informed choice regarding whether a terminal master's program might be a good option for you.

APPLYING TO GRADUATE SCHOOL

Applying to graduate school involves multiple steps over time, as well as several components that make up the application itself. In this section, we break down and review the application timeline and each of the required application materials.

The Application Timeline

We've provided a timeline for the application process, including steps for preparing your application materials, submitting your application, and preparing for and completing interviews (Figure 3.1). As you can see, there are a lot of

FIGURE 3.1. Graduate School Application and Interview Timeline

	Spring				Summer				Fall/Winter			
	Jan	Feb	Mar	Apr	May	Jun	Jul	Aug	Sep	Oct	Nov	Dec
Register for GRE					█							
Take/retake GRE						█	█	█	█	█		
Consider fit factors						█						
Look for programs						█	█					
Draft CV, personal statement							█	█				
Finalize program list									█			
Email faculty of interest									█			
Get feedback on CV and personal statement									█			
Request letters of rec									█			
Finalize application										█		
Submit application										█		
Do practice interviews											█	█
Attend actual interviews	█	█										
Await admissions decisions, select an offer			█	█								

Note. CV = curriculum vitae; GRE = Graduate Record Exam.

steps involved—the earlier you start, the less stressed you'll be as the application deadline looms.

Consider Fit Factors

In neuropsychology, graduate school forms a critical foundation for the other steps in your training journey. The majority of graduate programs entail a combination of clinical training, research, and didactics. Some grad programs are more research focused, some are more clinically focused, and some have an equal weighting between the two. This is something as an applicant that you will have to decide when weighing your personal *fit factors*, or the things that you take into consideration when weighing program factors (e.g., type, training philosophy, relative clinical vs. research emphasis, and so on) as well as individual factors (e.g., preferred geographic location, level of financial support, in line with clinical and research interests, opportunities to specialize in neuropsychology). Starting on page 13 of *The Neuropsychologist's Roadmap*, review Tip 3 to get a sense of some of the program-related fit factors you should be thinking about and help identify which ones are most important to you. Ask your mentors and current neuropsychology graduate students what factors were important to them when they were choosing among programs. If you don't know any current neuropsychology graduate students, you can email a doctoral program to ask if they would be willing to connect you. You could also connect with many of the neuropsychology trainees who are on social media platforms like X/Twitter (use the hashtag #neuropsychology to help you narrow down the search results).

You can consider shaping your own fit factors into a personalized ranking system, which you can apply to all programs of interest and help you identify which are the best suited for you. For example, in Table 3.1, our prospective applicant highly values programs that follow the scientist–practitioner model, has more than one neuropsychologist in the program who can serve as mentors, offers at least two neuropsychology practica, are in the mid-Atlantic region, and offer tuition waivers and guaranteed funding. By inputting and weighting the things they value, it creates a useful data point against which they can compare other graduate programs. Use the blank form on Table 3.2. Try inputting some of your own fit factors and use it as you review graduate school programs. You may also find that as you go through the application and interview process that you identify additional fit factors you had not thought of before.

TABLE 3.1. Fit Factors (Sample)

Fit factor category	Item and response			Score weights
Program factors	Program model	X	2	Scientist-practitioner
			1	Practitioner–scholar
			0	Clinical scientist
	Program faculty	X	2	More than one neuropsychologist
			1	One neuropsychologist
			0	No neuropsychologists
	Neuropsychology-specific practica	X	2	More than two practica in neuropsychology
			1	One or two practica in neuropsychology
			0	No practica in neuropsychology
Individual factors	Geographic location		4	Mid-Atlantic
			3	South/Southeast
			2	Midwest or Southwest
		X	1	West Coast or Northeast
			0	Other
	Level of financial support		2	Tuition waivers and guaranteed funding through grants and/or assistantships
		X	1	Tuition waivers but funding is not guaranteed
			0	No funding
	Total			8 points

TABLE 3.2. Fit Factors (Blank)

Fit factor category	Item and response			Score weights	
Program factors					
Individual factors					
	Total				

Do Your Homework

Tip 4 in Chapter 1 of *The Neuropsychologist's Roadmap*, "Applying and Getting Into Graduate School" provides several concrete ways for you to look up programs that provide training in neuropsychology. Another trick that we can pass on to you: If you use Microsoft Outlook, you can set up an alert so that any time you get an email containing the word "graduate school" you receive a notification. You can do this by following these instructions: (1) In Microsoft Outlook, select the home tab. (2) Select the "Rules" option, which falls underneath the "Move" section. (3) Select the "Manage Rules and Alerts" option, and then "New Rule" under the email tab. (4) From here, you can select any of the "Stay Up to Date" options. This includes playing a unique sound when one of these emails comes through.

As you review the programs, you will need some way of sorting through them to determine whether they are a potential fit. We recommend putting your thoughts to paper. Yes, actually write your thoughts on a sheet of paper. This will clarify quickly which sites are indeed a potential fit and which are not. It will also help you sketch out the information that becomes important in crafting your training goals at a given program. We've provided a worksheet (Table 3.3) that you can use to help you keep track of and organize information.

As you review neuropsychology doctoral program websites and brochures, fill out the table, devoting one row to each program so you can quickly get a sense of what the program has to offer. Remember, at this stage, you are just gathering information and learning about what different programs have to

TABLE 3.3. Program Review Worksheet (Blank)

Program name	APA or CPA accredited	SCN member or NP emphasis	Funding or financial support	Research interest match with faculty	No. of clinical practica sites	Location	Other

Note. APA = American Psychological Association; CPA = Canadian Psychological Association; NP = Neuropsychology; SCN = Society of Clinical Neuropsychology.

offer, and whether they could potentially be a good fit for you, so you'll probably want to cast a broad net. So even if you are thinking to yourself, "I'm not sure how I feel about living in the south," or "I don't see how this program could possibly have a good neuropsychology program—I've never heard of this university, and they're in the middle of nowhere!" put the program on the list anyway. Don't count out any programs based on preconceived ideas about location, cost, quality, etc. We'd recommend putting more than 15 programs on your list; the larger the list you start with, the more information you will have later as you whittle down and finalize the list of sites to which you will apply. Here are more specific instructions for how to fill out the table; we've added columns for you based on what we think are some factors that set programs apart, and are important for you to consider.

- **APA/Canadian Psychological Association accredited:** Indicate whether the site is APA accredited, not accredited, or awaiting accreditation. Be cautious about nonaccredited programs; attending one will make it harder for you when you go on to apply for internship programs, postdoctoral programs, and board certification.

- **Society of Clinical Neuropsychology (SCN) member/major area of study:** Write down whether the program is listed in the training directory of the SCN and/or whether clinical neuropsychology is offered as a major area of study, an emphasis, experience, or exposure. This information will help you determine the degree of training intensity within clinical neuropsychology (i.e., the education and training opportunities available specifically in clinical neuropsychology). A program that offers neuropsychology as a major area of study or emphasis will make it easier for you to obtain neuropsychology-specific internships.

- **Funding/financial support:** Is funding guaranteed? If not, what percentage of students are funded? Also write down the average stipend, the range of stipends, how much tuition is every year, and whether there is a tuition waiver.

- **Match with research interests:** Review the list of faculty members in the department and their research interests. Write down the faculty members with whom you have matching research interests. Typically, faculty members have a blurb on the website or brochure describing their research interests. If this information is not readily available to you, you may need to do some extra research by looking up their recently published research papers.

- **Number of neuropsychologists:** Review the list of faculty members and write down how many of them are neuropsychologists.

- **Number of clinical practica sites:** Write down how many internal and external practica are offered by the program and how many of the practica are neuropsychology specific. To be competitive for an internship with specialization in neuropsychology, it's crucial that you have clinical experience in neuropsychological assessment. So the more neuropsychology specific practica available in that program, the easier it will be when it comes down to applying for internships.

- **Location:** In what city/state/province is the site located?

- **Other:** Here you can add any other fit factors that are important to you that have not been listed. For instance, some programs are structured in a way that they allow a minor area of study, and you can use this opportunity to acquire specialty skills (e.g., computer skills, specialty neuroscience, or computational methods).

Now that you've prioritized the programs that fit most with what you are looking for, and you have a list, it's time to start the application process.

Essential Elements of Your Application

For most applications, you will need to submit a personal statement, a CV (curriculum vitae), a copy of your undergraduate transcript, and at least three letters of recommendation. Some may also require the general Graduate Record Exams (GREs), psychology GREs, and a writing sample. Although the elements of the application may be the same, each program will have its own requirements for the format, structure, and content. You want to demonstrate that you are detail-oriented and conscientious in your application; that means reading and following all instructions pertaining to the application.

We recommend that you use a system where you can keep track of all the requirements, stay organized, and have the information readily available in one place. See Table 3.4, which we've provided for you to use while doing this. You can see that you'd want to fill out this table once you have narrowed down your site list and be detailed as you fill it out (because some sites will want specific information included in the application, like in the cover letter, for example). Remember to include details regarding the content (e.g., suggestions of what your cover letter should include) and format (e.g., word count, file type) of different elements of your application, as well as information about how you will submit the application (e.g., where to send your materials, when it is due).

The summer months are good times to begin putting your application together and create first drafts of all your application elements. This allows for plenty of time for you to solicit and receive feedback from your mentors in the months of September and October and then to complete your revisions in the month of November before submission.

Emailing Faculty Members

Although this is not a necessary step, we would highly recommend that you email the faculty members you are interested in working with in the months of September and October. Tip 4 in Chapter 1 of *The Neuropsychologist's Roadmap* provides some helpful do's and don'ts for this email and why this step is helpful. We've provided a template email for you to follow (Exhibit 3.1). Now let's talk about each element of your application in a little bit more detail.

TABLE 3.4. Application Requirements for Graduate Programs (Blank)

Program name	Deadline	Fee	Desired GRE scores	Requires personal statement?	No. of letters of recommendation	Requires transcript?	Requires writing sample?	Requires resume or CV?	Other

Note. CV = curriculum vitae; GRE = Graduate Record Exam.

EXHIBIT 3.1

Sample Email to Faculty

Dear Dr. XX,

My name is [Your Name] and I am reaching out because I will be applying to the Psychology program at XX this upcoming fall, and I am interested in joining your lab as a graduate student.

I am currently a research assistant at YY, and under the guidance of Dr. YY [Current Mentor's Name], I have been working on [Brief description of your Job and/or research area]. I am specifically interested in [description of your research interest, constructs, methods]. I find your work on [Faculty member's research interests] deeply interesting, particularly [Specific details about that faculty member's recent work].

I am inquiring as to whether you are accepting PhD candidates for the upcoming application cycle. I have attached my CV as a reference. Thank you in advance for your time and consideration, and I look forward to hearing more about your work.

Sincerely,

[Your Name]

Dear Dr. Patricia,

My name is Evelyn Blake and I am reaching out because I will be applying to the Psychology program at Green Gables University this upcoming fall, and I am interested in joining your lab as a graduate student.

I am currently a research assistant at Avonlea Technical College, and under the guidance of Dr. Matthew, I have been working on a study elucidating gender differences in cognitive skills in children with various genetic disorders. I am deeply interested in your line of research work following young adults with neurofibromatosis type 2, particularly your investigation using functional neuroimaging methods to elucidate the neurobiological networks that can underlie attention deficits in this population.

I am inquiring as to whether you are accepting PhD candidates for the upcoming application cycle. I have attached my CV as a reference. Thank you in advance for your time and consideration, and I look forward to hearing more about your work.

Sincerely,

[Your Name]

Your Curriculum Vitae

According to a review by Barclay Simpson (2023), employers spend 30 seconds at most (and sometimes as little as 6 seconds) reviewing an applicant's resume. While data do not exist for the academic arena, we think that figure is not likely to change by much. So it's important that your CV be visually streamlined, consistent, well structured, and with only the most relevant content to allow reviewers to locate the information they need quickly to decide whether to extend an interview offer. You can see a range of CV tips in Table 3.5, and we have even provided a sample template for you to follow (Exhibit 3.2).

TABLE 3.5. Curriculum Vitae (CV) Tips

Do	Don't
✓ Use clear and succinct headers.	✗ Use lots of font embellishments like bolding, italics, and underlining. Simple is better.
✓ Put information you want to highlight toward the beginning. For example, if it's a research-focused program, then consider putting your list of presentations and publications ahead of your clinical experience.	✗ Use inconsistent spacing or formatting throughout.
✓ Use a simple, clear font such as Arial, Verdana, Calibri, Times New Roman, or Georgia. Depending on the font, its size should be no less than 10 points and no larger than 12 points (excepting headers).	✗ Organize information by oldest first. It is better to place more recent information first, followed by older in sequential order.
✓ Include your name and page number at the bottom of all pages in your CV.	✗ Be too text-heavy because this creates more work (and increases visual fatigue) on the part of the reviewer. Consider replacing walls of text with bullet points. For example, under clinical rotations, you might wish to include bullet points that specify the name and credentials of your supervisor(s), type of training experience (e.g., pediatric neuropsychology private practice), major populations (e.g., dementia, movement disorders, epilepsy), and primary activities (e.g., therapy, clinical interview, testing, scoring, report writing).
✓ Position dates to the left-hand side. Dates should be presented in "Month Year—Month Year" or "Year" format.	
✓ Double check any page breaks, and if needed, adjust spacing so you're not left with hanging information across pages.	
✓ Present publications and presentations as numbered lists, and be sure to underline or bold your name in each citation to make it more visible to your reviewer.	✗ Include poster publication info in both the poster and publication sections. This looks like you are padding your CV. If you happen to have a poster published in a journal, include that information in the same citation as the poster.

Your Personal Statement or Cover Letter

The way to make your application stand out is to demonstrate how you would be a good fit for a particular research mentor and/or program. People reviewing your application will know if you wrote a generic personal statement and sent the same copy to all the graduate programs you are applying to. There are no shortcuts here. You will need to personalize each cover letter/personal statement such that your reviewers can easily answer the following questions: Can I and this program help this applicant meet their goals? Is this applicant a good fit for my research lab and this program? Use the worksheet in Table 3.6 to help you brainstorm and ultimately articulate why you would be a good fit for that research mentor, program, or lab. You'll use this information when you are writing your personal statement. Fill out each column based on the following:

- **Experiences I have:** List all the clinical and research experiences you have, including the populations you have worked with, clinical skills you have developed, the research questions you have been exploring, and the methods you've learned to explore those questions.

EXHIBIT 3.2

Curriculum Vitae Template

CURRICULUM VITAE

CLARK KENT, BS

CONTACT INFORMATION

1438 Lois Lane
Smallville, KS 123456
Phone: (101) 123-1234
Email: Jane.Doe@Smallville.edu
Web: www.linkedin.com/in/janedoe

EDUCATION

8/2019–Present	PhD, Clinical Psychology (neuropsychology focus) Smallville University; Smallville, KS Dissertation: The relationship between increased brain volume and reading this workbook Chair: Perry White, PhD
8/2013–5/2017	BS, Psychology (magna cum laude) Krypton College Cumulative GPA: 3.59/4.00 Major GPA: 3.99/4.00

AWARDS, HONORS, & RECOGNITION

2017	Outstanding Undergraduate Award, Krypton College Dept of Psychology
2016	Presentation Award, Smallville Academy of Sciences conference
2014–2017	Dean's List, Krypton College

LEADERSHIP & SERVICE

10/2019–Present	Chair, Neuropsychology Interest Group, Smallville University
8/2018–7/2019	Student Rep, Dept of Psychology Committee, Smallville University
08/2016–05/2017	President, Psi Chi Chapter, Krypton College
01/2011–07/2013	Volunteer, Smallville Chapter, Alzheimer's Association

PROFESSIONAL MEMBERSHIPS

2013–Present	Student Affiliate, Metropolis Society for Neuropsychology
2015–2017	Psi Chi Honor Society

CLINICAL TRAINING

8/2016–Present	The Daily Planet Clinic Department of Psychiatry, Smallville University Medical Center; Smallville, KS Supervisor(s): Perry White, PhD, Arthur Curry, PsyD, ABPP-CN Training Activities: Worked as a psychometrist, and performed test administration and scoring as part of comprehensive neuropsychological evaluations. Additional activities included collecting and organizing data for clinical research purposes. Exposed to a range of populations including Alzheimer's disease, Parkinson's disease, traumatic brain injury, epilepsy, stroke, and psychiatric conditions.

(continues)

EXHIBIT 3.2

Curriculum Vitae Template (*Continued*)

REFEREED PUBLICATIONS

1. <u>Kent, C.</u>, & White, P. (2019). Efficacy of kryptonite in the treatment of mild cognitive impairment. *The Journal of The Metropolis Society for Neuropsychology*, *33*(1), 159–172.
2. Themyscira, D., Curry, A., Stone, V., <u>Kent, C.</u>, & White, P. (2018). Working memory and kryptonite: A dose–response relationship. *Atlantean Communications, under review.*

NONREFEREED PUBLICATIONS

1. <u>Kent, C.</u>, & Stone, V. (2017). Kryptonite: A new horizon in the treatment of brain disorders? *Smallville University Magazine, 10*, 12–15.

PRESENTATIONS & PUBLISHED ABSTRACTS

1. <u>Kent, C.</u>, & White, P. (2018). Efficacy of kryptonite in the treatment of mild cognitive impairment. Poster presented at the Metropolis Society for Neuropsychology conference; Metropolis, KS. *The Journal of The Metropolis Society for Neuropsychology, 32*(3), 159.

TABLE 3.6. Personal Statement Brainstorming Worksheet

Experiences I have	My training goals and long-term career goals	What does the program offer?	What do I bring to the table?

- **My training goals and long-term career goals:** In this column, write down your short- and long-term goals. Brainstorm answers to these questions: What clinical populations do I want to work with? What skills do I want to learn in clinical work and in research? What research topics and questions do I want to explore? What do I want to be doing in 10 years? What type of setting do I want to work in? You can obviously change your mind in the future, but you want to have some clear goals in mind right now.

- **What does the site offer:** Review the program website, browse through the faculty members' page summarizing the work they have been doing, and read through recent papers from those labs. Ideally, you've done some of the legwork already when you came up with a list of graduate programs you wanted to apply to. But expand on this by writing down the opportunities that are offered at that program and lab, including the populations you might work with; the clinical practica available; the research aims, questions, and topics being explored; and the research methods being used. We recommend creating a separate bullet point for each faculty member to help you keep track of which research topics are specific to that person.

- **What do I bring to the table:** Review what you wrote in Columns 1 and 2, and think about how that might fit in with what you wrote in Column 3. What could you, with your unique clinical and research experiences, bring to the table at that site? Is there anything you can add to what they are already doing? You don't need to be a perfect fit! But applicants are typically more compelling if their future training and career goals broadly align with what the site has to offer and if there is a logical connection between the experiences they have had and the topic of research being explored in the lab. The more explicit you are as to what you can bring to the table and how good a fit you are, the better, so take your time thinking about this. Spend time on this step—you'll use this content when you write your letter.

Letters of Recommendation

All the programs to which you'll apply will require letters of recommendation. Most graduate school programs ask for three letters. Some applicants wonder whether they should submit more, and—as a general rule—we strongly advise that you do not submit any more letters than the site requires. The last thing you want to do in your application is give the appearance that you are unable to follow directions!

Who should be your letter writers? As a whole, these letters should be able to speak to your academic, research, clinical, and interpersonal dimensions. Brainstorm the different people in your life who could serve as recommenders. Your reviewers should be able to glean a picture of your academic, clinical (neuropsychology and general), research, and interpersonal skills. Don't worry if no single person can speak to all these skills in a single letter, but you will want to prioritize the individuals who can speak to your qualities in multiple domains.

If you are finding that there are some gaps in coverage and it is early enough in the application timeline for you to address them, you may want to prioritize building relationships with people who could help write a letter that speaks to that domain. See if there are any ways you can leverage relationships you already have. For instance, if you are taking a course with an instructor and they can speak to your academic skills (but nothing else), could you attend office hours so they can speak to some of your interpersonals? Could you ask them to mentor you on a thesis research project so they can speak to your research skills? If you find that you have significant gaps and that more than two domains will not be addressed by any of your letter writers, then you may want to engage in some self-reflection and determine whether you are truly ready to apply for graduate school at this time.

When you have decided on your letter writers, give them plenty of time to author the letter. We recommend asking at least 1 month in advance. We find it helpful when candidates prepare a packet that we can reference during this letter-writing process. Consider including some or all of the following items in the packet:

- **Program listing:** For each program, include the full program name (with department if applicable), the name and credentials of the program training director, instructions on to whom the letter should be sent (and by what means), and clear due dates. It also helps to include submission instructions (e.g., via email? Web portal?). Include the actual email or weblink if applicable, or note that the writer should expect an email containing a weblink. Since you will be applying to multiple sites, we recommend providing all this information in an organized way (see Table 3.7).

- **Shared experience list:** We find that it is also helpful if applicants include a bullet-point list (briefly) outlining experiences they've shared with that specific person. Did they teach one or more of your classes? Did you publish or present anything together? Did you work together clinically? Were you a teaching assistant for them?

- **Curriculum vitae (CV):** You should also include an updated version of your CV.

- **Letter of interest:** It may be helpful to include a sample letter from your application, because this should include clear goals for your future that your letter writer may wish to reference.

One last bit of advice: It is kind to remind. Being supervisors and letter-writers ourselves, we find it helpful to receive a reminder at the 1-week mark, assuming that the letter has not been written yet. In the reminder, include the due date and information on who the letter will be going to (i.e., program/training director name and email, or weblink if relevant).

Finalizing Your Site List

September and October are good months to finalize the list of graduate programs to which you intend to apply. Use the fit factors worksheet you

TABLE 3.7. Instructions for Letters of Recommendation Writers

Date *Deadline*	Program name *Include department and institution*	Program director *Include name and credentials*	Special instructions *Specify submission via email or web portal*

completed to help you finalize your list, prioritizing the programs that have higher totals. How many programs should be on your final list? In our survey, respondents felt that applicants should apply to no fewer than eight and no more than 15 programs (on average), although there was a little bit of variability. All in all, we think you are safe applying to somewhere between 10 to 15 programs. We have a section later in this chapter with more information on what makes a competitive applicant, which can help you decide whether you should lean more toward the lower or higher end. So, for instance, if you have a lot of the experiences and qualities that people reviewing graduate school applicants are looking for, you can probably lean more toward applying to 10 programs. If you find that you are missing some key experiences and feel a little bit more worried about your prospects, maybe lean more toward applying to 15 (or more) programs.

Final Check Before Submitting

There is absolutely nothing worse than that sinking feeling you get when you realize 2 seconds after clicking the "submit application" button that you submitted the wrong cover letter or misspelled the name of the faculty member with whom you most want to work. One way to limit mistakes is to keep your submission materials organized. We recommend that you create a folder for each program you are applying to and label each document with the name of the program. So, for instance, if you are applying to Middle Earth University, the individual files in the Middle Earth University folder could be as follows: Middle Earth University_Cover Letter.pdf, Middle Earth University_CV. pdf, Middle Earth University_Transcript.pdf, and Middle Earth University_ WritingSample.doc. This will help you ensure that you are uploading the correct files for your application.

MAKING YOURSELF COMPETITIVE

In our survey, we asked neuropsychologists who are currently or have previously been involved in the review of graduate school applications what makes applications stand out. Specifically, what should applicants do, and what sorts of things should they avoid? There were common themes in their responses, which we've provided in Table 3.8. We also asked our survey respondents to choose (up to) five factors that are most important to them when reviewing an application to a graduate program.

There were four clear factors that were considered the most important. Having a strong research interest fit and having clinical experiences in neuropsychology were both tied, with 65% of neuropsychologists saying that these were in their top five factors. Next was the strength of the letters of recommendation. In our experience, a lukewarm letter can really sink an application; make sure to ask all your letter-writers whether they would be able to write you a strong letter of application. And then 50% of neuropsychologists taking

TABLE 3.8. Application Do's and Don'ts

Do	Don't
✓ Highlight previous relevant experiences (specifically research, clinical work, and educational experiences), future goals, and fit with the specific program.	✗ Submit vague, generic, and unpolished personal statements.
✓ Articulate how working in a specific lab or a specific program will support your future goals very clearly. Make sure your responses are tailored to that faculty/ program. Integrate your experience with the research of the lab to which you are applying to tell a story about who you want to be in 10 years.	✗ Submit application components that are not proofread. Often programs are getting many applicants that look similar on paper, so small copyediting errors can put you below someone of similar caliber.
✓ Be willing to suggest future areas of inquiry that relate to the faculty member's work and are of interest to the applicant.	✗ Self-disclose without a specific purpose. Personal anecdotes are welcome but use them sparingly and for a specific purpose. Self-disclosures are most effective when they shed light on why you are interested in a topic or when they explain a part of your application that otherwise looks like a weakness. Anecdotes to avoid include talking about your personal psychiatric history as your reason for applying to a doctorate program; discussing how you were pre-med but then failed a class so now you are applying to psychology; saying you want to help people; providing poignant vignettes about how you once helped somebody, especially a family member or friend; say that you came to psychology because you didn't know what else to do.
✓ If you have experience in advanced statistics or real programming experience (e.g., MATLAB, R, Python), highlight this in your personal statement.	
✓ Express your enthusiasm for the field of neuropsychology, your intellectual curiosity, and love of learning.	
✓ Use your personal statement to convey something that cannot be found elsewhere in the application to allow the programs to get to know you.	
✓ Highlight motivation, work ethic, and clear desire/commitment for a career in neuropsychology.	✗ Overstate or exaggerate your experiences, accomplishments, or qualifications.
✓ If you are fluent in another language, highlight this in your personal statement.	✗ Misspell/use incorrect faculty or university/college names.
✓ Highlight if you have exposure to neuropsychological testing experience, and report writing experience.	✗ Equate neuropsychology with testing psychology.
	✗ Wait until the last minute to complete applications. When feeling exhausted or rushed, it's easy to make careless errors, and unexpected problems can ensue that can hold up a potential mentor's review of your application.
	✗ State a disinterest in any area of training the site requires.

our survey indicated that a diverse applicant and/or an applicant who demonstrates a commitment to diversity is considered one of their top five factors when reviewing an application. A commitment to diversity can be demonstrated both through the quality of your past experiences on your CV (research, clinical) and through your personal statement if you can genuinely speak to your passion and commitment to diversity. A little less than half of our sample indicated that having peer-reviewed publications in scholarly journals would be seen as a top five factor. We take this to mean that if you have a publication, it is seen as positive by many, but you also shouldn't be too worried if you don't have any publications before submitting your application.

Related to that point, we asked a series of questions about research productivity—specifically, how many publications, oral presentations, and/or posters would be expected of a competitive applicant. When it comes to publications, a majority of our respondents (58%) indicated that they expect an average of one publication; 21% of our respondents said they don't expect any publications of a competitive applicant, and 26% said they expected at least two publications. When it comes to oral presentations, a majority (53%) didn't expect any oral presentations of a competitive applicant, while 26% expected one, and 21% expected at least two oral presentations. And when it came to posters, a majority of our survey respondents (74%) indicated they expected at least two posters of a competitive applicant, while 16% indicated that they expected just one poster, and 11% indicated they expected no posters. All in all, we take this to mean that if you want to be competitive for a PhD program, you should have at least one publication, at least two posters, and you shouldn't worry if you don't have any oral presentations. This is not to say that you won't get into graduate school if you don't have these numbers, but these are good benchmarks to strive for if you want to be a competitive applicant (to a PhD program; PsyD programs have less of an emphasis on research, so you won't need these numbers to be a competitive applicant).

Another note: we know that some of you may not have ready access to neuropsychology research lab experience but were still productive with your posters and publications in other types of labs. We specifically asked neuropsychologists how they would view it if an applicant had posters, presentations, or publications but none of them were related to neuropsychology, neuroscience, or neurology topics. As mentioned before, 65% of our sample indicated that they would still view this experience positively—that is, any experience in publishing or presenting is a meaningful experience—and 25% said they were neutral (i.e., didn't matter to them). Only 10% of our survey respondents stated that they would view this experience negatively. If this applies to you, we highly recommend that you devote some space in your personal statement explaining why you are pivoting from one area of research to another.

We also want to highlight the factors that were not selected as the top five most important factors in an application. None of our sample indicated that psychology GRE scores, volunteering experience, or barriers that applicants had to overcome were in their top five factors. And only 5% indicated that leadership experience was seen as a top five factor for them. To be clear, we are not saying that these experiences are worthless or undesired. We provide these statistics to help inform you as to which factors are broadly considered the most important by neuropsychologists reading an application. We hope this will help you focus your experiences in your undergrad and postbachelor's years, and also emphasize specific pieces of your application to make sure you stand out.

INTERVIEWING AT GRADUATE SCHOOL PROGRAMS

If you have received one or more offers for an interview, congratulations! You'll want to give your interview as much attention as your application. In our survey, we asked neuropsychologists what advice they have for applicants regarding interviews, as well as questions applicants should ask during their interviews for graduate school. There were quite a few common themes in their responses, which we've organized for you here.

- **Tip 1: Think about the fit.** One survey respondent said, "It cannot be understated how important fit is for both the program and trainee. Treat your interviews as an opportunity to explore this and to demonstrate to the program why you would fit there." Remember: You are interviewing the program as much as the program is interviewing you. Graduate school is hard, and you will be miserable if the program, mentor, and/or research aren't a good fit for you and your goals.

- **Tip 2: Prepare and practice.** As one of our survey respondents wrote, "Prepare beforehand so you can have substantive conversations with faculty members during your interview. It communicates interest and motivation." Broadly, you will prepare by doing your homework on the program and the mentor; preparing questions to ask; and preparing answers to some common questions in advance so you can be polished, specific, and thoughtful when you are in the interview. Here are our recommendations for how you can prepare and practice.

  ✓ *Be familiar with research being done in the lab by the mentor.* Typically, sites will provide a list of the faculty that you will be interviewing with. As written by one of our respondents: "You will want to demonstrate that you've read, understood, and processed the general aims of the lab and how they mesh with your training needs and goals." We recommend that you review the faculty member's website, social media, and some of their recent publications to get a sense of their research interests and recent findings.

  ✓ *Read through the program materials.* Be familiar with the program broadly as well. What kinds of practica are available? What type of training model do they have?

  ✓ *Prepare questions. Lots and lots of questions.* Try to have common questions regarding clinical training, research experiences, mentoring, internship and postdoc statistics, and work–life balance so you can compare data effectively across different training sites. But try not to ask questions that are easily answered by looking at the program's website or faculty member's lab website. If you do this, you risk looking unprepared. You will want to prepare questions for faculty members (see Exhibit 3.3 for some sample questions you can ask faculty members). On that note, try not to run out of questions, even if this is your last interview of a long and exhausting day! It can signal disinterest and can be viewed

EXHIBIT 3.3

Sample Interview Questions

Sample Questions for and About Faculty

- What is your mentorship style?
- What attracted you to this program/this job?
- What is the supervision or training model in your lab?
- What is the funding availability in your lab?
- What flexibility do students have to work on projects related to their interests? I see the lab has been doing X, Y, and Z; are those areas of focus in the next few years?
- What projects are you are working on currently?
- What are some future directions you feel the lab is headed in? (And be ready to continue this conversation about how you might be a part of those new directions).
- What types of research do you hope to do over the next 5 years? or Where do you see your research headed in the next 5 years?
- What qualities and characteristics do your most successful graduate students have?
- How should I prepare for entering a doctoral program before stepping foot on campus?
- What are you looking for in a graduate student?
- What are some barriers to students completing the program in a timely manner?

Sample Questions for and About the Program

- What is the split between clinical and research training? or How much emphasis is on research versus clinical training?
- How does this program balance the broad and general training in clinical (or counseling) psychology with specialty training in clinical neuropsychology?
- How does your curriculum align with modern competency models in clinical neuropsychology?
- How does your program contribute to a trainee's preparation to be a board-certified clinical neuropsychologist?
- What is the best part about this program? What is the most challenging part about this program?
- What are the strengths of the program?
- What types of practicum placements do your students typically secure?
- What are your former students doing now? What sorts of research or future jobs do your former students have now?
- Where do trainees go after completing the program?
- What types of patient populations are seen by students in their practica?
- What does the program do to support diverse students or students from nontraditional backgrounds?

Sample Questions for Graduate Students

- How much of your time is devoted to coursework versus clinical versus teaching versus research?
- What does a typical week look like for you?
- Are students typically able to support themselves on the stipend, or do they need to take out loans?
- What is one thing you wish you would have known about the program before you came?

EXHIBIT 3.3

Sample Interview Questions (*Continued*)

- What is one thing you wish you would have known about your research mentor before you came?
- What is one thing you wish you would have known about this city before you came?
- Do you have time to take vacations during the year?
- How do you spend your weekends?

Questions You Should Be Prepared to Answer

- Tell me about your research interests, aka the "elevator pitch."
- Why do you want to become a neuropsychologist?
- Tell me about the clinical experiences you have had.
- Tell me about the research experiences you've had so far.
- What are your goals for graduate school? What are your career goals?
- Why us? That is, what about this program in particular interests you and would make you good a fit?
- What can you offer to this program? What can you offer to this lab?
- What ideas do you have for a master's thesis or doctoral dissertation?
- What types of new collaborations and new directions could you foresee for our lab?

negatively. Also, you will want to prepare questions for current graduate students (see Exhibit 3.3 for some sample questions). Most programs will provide a time for you to speak to current graduate students, whether that's on the interview day or a social event within the interview period. If the program doesn't provide a time, ask whether you can contact current graduate students to ask them questions about the program. It is very unusual for a program to be unwilling to let you speak to current graduate students and could potentially be a red flag. Current graduate students are an excellent source of information, and this is another opportunity for you to ask questions that will help you see whether the program would be a good fit for you. Many of the questions listed under the sample questions for the mentor/faculty member and questions to ask about the program can also be asked of current graduate students, and it's a great way to find out whether faculty and graduate students share similar views on the program. Also, assume that you are being evaluated and remain professional in all your interactions, even if they tell you that you are not being evaluated.

✓ *Prepare answers.* As one survey respondent wrote, "Faculty members want to see an applicant who has specific and thought-through responses." Having a trusted mentor, friend, or someone in the career center conduct a mock interview with you will also be very helpful—this way, you can get feedback as to the quality and content of your responses and whether you are able to get your meaning across concisely and succinctly. Another note: While you want to look prepared and confident, you also don't want to appear overrehearsed/robotic. See Exhibit 3.3

for some sample questions that you may be asked. Another note: Your interviewer will likely wish to know why you are interested in the field. You want your answer to be authentic, and therefore, self-disclosing something that stimulated your interest, imagination, or curiosity in the field is fine. We encourage you to refresh your memory by reviewing Table 3.8. in the "don't" column regarding self-disclosure and topics to avoid.

- **Tip 3: Find ways to manage anxiety and fatigue.** Interviews typically start early in the morning and extend into the late afternoon, and there may even be other social events set up within the interview period for you to meet with current graduate students. You will meet with many people—faculty, staff, and graduate students. You may be asked to walk around the building or across campus for a tour. What this means is that interview days are long, fatiguing, and anxiety-provoking. One neuropsychologist wrote, "It's nerve-wracking to do interviews, and interviewers can tell if you are managing the anxiety well or not." Another neuropsychologist recommended, "Be prepared for a long day and practice fatigue/mood management techniques so you can present consistently across interviewers." You know best what helps you manage your anxiety and fatigue. Is it a quick 5-minute walking break? A deep-breathing exercise? Listening to your favorite song in between interviews? Talking to other applicants about hobbies or interests? Be deliberate and consciously make choices so you can engage in your fatigue and mood management strategies during the interview day.

- **Tip 4: Show your personality.** As one survey respondent wrote, "Most faculty members want to see an applicant who seems like they would fit well into the larger group since most graduate programs are essentially small communities where others have to work for you for 4 or more years." As we've said before, fit is so important—and that extends to personality fit. Faculty members will also assess whether you could mesh well with the lab and program.

- **Tip 5: Be genuine and authentic.** One survey respondent advised, "[Ask questions] that [you] genuinely want the answer to; don't ask questions just to fill time or because you think you have to." We emphasized earlier that it's important not to run out of questions. However, it's also equally important that you are asking questions that you genuinely want answers to. It will be obvious to your interviewers if you are asking questions just to ask questions. If you find that you are not genuinely eager to talk to faculty members or fellow students, it could be a sign that you are not a good fit for that site.

- **Tip 6: Demonstrate traits that will help you succeed in graduate school.** These were the common ones that were listed by the neuropsychologists who responded to our survey: enthusiasm, curiosity, compassion, genuineness, empathy, warmth, cultural humility, and intellectual humility.

Remember, you are applying to a clinical psychology program, and these are core competencies necessary for the degree. Relatedly, one neuropsychologist noted, "Remember that everyone you meet could be part of the interview process. This includes students, staff, and people you meet in the hallway. Be kind and polite in all interactions." You could be the most accomplished applicant with strong research and clinical experiences, but a poor, unprofessional interaction with anyone involved in the interview process could automatically strike you from consideration from the program.

- **Tip 7: If you have a telephone or video interview, take extra time to test your setup.** More and more interviews are moving to telephone and video conference formats, which is great! You don't have to worry about travel costs or cancellations or delays that could prevent you from making it to the interview. We recommend that you still dress professionally (even if the interview is over the phone—you never know if someone will unexpectedly ask you to hop onto a video call). Test your setup and internet connection well before the interview starts. One clinical neuropsychologist advised, "You might be surprised how distracting your office bookshelves are or you may find that the lighting is better in one place over another. Although these are small things, they can distract interviewers from focusing on your answers and all the great things you could bring to their program." Take note of anything else that could be distracting in the room—the chirp of a fire detector that needs its battery changed? An office phone that could ring at any minute? We also know that although it may ease your anxiety to have a written script of answers to common questions in front of you, your interviewer will be able to tell if you are reading from a script. Try to avoid doing this by practicing your responses. It will help your answers look authentic rather than overrehearsed.

- **Tip 8: Take written notes with the answers to your questions and how you felt about the program.** We recommend that you write down all this information as quickly as you can after the interview day. If you have time during breaks to jot down some notes, that works too. If you are fortunate to have more than one interview, you will find that this information will start to blur together. Having a written account of answers to your questions and your impressions will ensure that you have a more accurate recall of that site.

- **Tip 9: Send thank you emails—but also listen to programs that explicitly tell you not to send them.** To some faculty members, thank you emails can mean a lot because it demonstrates interest and enthusiasm in the program and lab. To other faculty members, thank you notes make absolutely no difference. Writing thank you notes is not a requirement, but it can be nice to do, especially if you are genuinely interested in the program. If you choose to write a thank you note, keep your communication short, sweet, and professional. If you ask any follow-up questions, make sure the question hasn't already been answered before in the program materials

---

EXHIBIT 3.4

Sample Email to Faculty Postinterview

Dear Dr. [Faculty Member's Last Name],

I wanted to say a quick thank you for the opportunity to interview at your program and speak to you about your research. It was wonderful to get to talk with you about the study you are in the process of completing and about the ongoing projects in the lab. I had a fantastic time visiting. I also enjoyed the friendly and supportive vibe from your current graduate students, and I feel that your lab would be an excellent fit for my research interests. Thank you!

Sincerely,

[Your Name]

---

or otherwise and that you are genuinely interested in the answer. There is one very important exception to sending thank you emails: Some programs will explicitly tell applicants not to send them. Follow their instructions! Sending an email may give off the impression that you are inflexible or that you do not follow directions, and this is not an impression you want to make. We provide a sample email you can adapt for your own use in Exhibit 3.4.

In Exhibit 3.5, we provide the interview factors that survey respondents considered most and least important when interviewing applicants. When reviewing their responses, it's clear that it really is all about fit—clinical fit, research fit, and personality fit.

EXHIBIT 3.5

Survey Results: Ranked Interview Factors

Top-Ranked Factors (Most Important First)

- Demonstrates clinical fit/promise
- Demonstrates research fit/promise
- Demonstrates personality fit with faculty, supervisors, and other students
- Being well prepared for the interview (e.g., high-quality questions and responses to interview questions)

Bottom-Ranked Factors (Least Important First)

- Workplace-appropriate appearance and attire
- Nonverbal behaviors and mannerisms
- Quality of responses to standardized interview questions
- Quality of general verbal interaction

TIPS FOR INTERNATIONAL APPLICANTS

For those of you who are applying from a country outside of the United States, we also gathered some helpful advice from survey respondents. Here are some of their suggestions: (a) Apply to programs at schools with a good international student office; (b) know as much as you can about the snags inherent in the system that may affect visa status, funding, and time constraints; (c) understand American training pathways and how they are similar and different from models of training that non-U.S. mentors may have experienced; and (d) understand how being an international applicant may impact practicum/internship opportunities (for instance, you will not be able to apply for internships at the Department of Veterans Affairs).

And when it comes to your graduate school application and interviews, here is what we think you should emphasize:

- Demonstrate what unique qualities you can add to the program (e.g., bilingual assessments, diversity, different perspectives).

- Writing samples would be important to demonstrate English proficiency, which can be helpful to manage all the coursework and writing demands in graduate training.

- If your primary language is not English, be prepared to address questions about your facility with English.

- Emphasize available social support, and if you have none, attempt to communicate how you plan on establishing support if accepted.

- Demonstrate sufficient familiarity and openness to be able to work with clients and colleagues from various backgrounds within the United States or other immigrants.

- Communicate that you are an international applicant to their site so they can determine their ability to support you financially within the parameters of their funding sources.

There are also a number of financial considerations. Understand how graduate school may impact costs because funding opportunities may be fewer or may have more barriers. Here are some ways you may be impacted:

- International students can't take federal loans.

- Being a non-U.S. citizen/green card holder means you can't apply for federal grants.

- You may have to take more classes for full-time status.

- You may have to rely on teaching fellowships.

- There may be language barriers for various practicum/funded opportunities. For instance, a program may offer testing for funding but may require that you do not have an accent.

To compensate for this, try to find out about on-campus work opportunities and financial aid opportunities. Consider inquiring about the past success of international students in the program and if they faced any challenges that impacted them. Ask about the program's experience with international students, including years to graduate and match rates for internship and postdoc (this can help gauge a program's level of support). Finally, ask whether the site can hire you based on their organization's hiring requirements.

AFTER INTERVIEWS

The procedure for the postinterview process is outlined in detail in Tips 11 and 12 (pp. 28–30) of *The Neuropsychologist's Roadmap*. You may also find it helpful to review another resource, the *Insider's Guide to Graduate Programs in Clinical and Counseling Psychology* (Norcross & Seyette, 2022). Our recommendation at this stage is to be deliberate in self-care activities. This stage can be even more anxiety-provoking than other stages of this process because there is nothing you can do to affect the outcome. Schedule activities that will help distract you and activate your support network. If you hear back and accept an offer, congratulations! If you don't get admitted, that's okay. It's time to self-reflect, review the strengths and weaknesses in your application (ideally with a mentor), and come up with an action plan to make you a stronger applicant for the next year. We have provided a worksheet where you can create an action plan to help you better prepare over the next year (see Table 3.9).

LOOKING AHEAD: SUCCESS IN GRADUATE SCHOOL

We know, we know. You just got into graduate school and the last thing you want to be thinking about is internship, which is a good 4 to 6 years away at this point. The first year of your graduate program will likely emphasize coursework and getting set up with research, but after that, you are going to start doing clinical work. If you are in a program that offers an emphasis in neuropsychology, then your program has likely already set up good-quality neuropsychology practica and can provide mentorship that is specifically tailored toward a career in neuropsychology. If this is not the case, the onus will be on you to seek out the experiences you will need to be competitive for an internship in neuropsychology. We recommend that you read *The Neuropsychologist's Roadmap* (especially the chapters related to preparing for internship and postdoctoral fellowship, as well as the chapters related to foundational competencies in neuropsychology), as well as Chapter 4 in this workbook related to preparation for applying to internship. We provide some benchmarks for the number of posters, publications, assessment/intervention hours, and reports that are typical for a competitive applicant in neuropsychology. You can use these as your endpoints. Keep track of how you are progressing toward these benchmarks every year and use this information to help focus your efforts for

TABLE 3.9. Action Plan

Application weaknesses	Goals to accomplish for next time	How to accomplish each goal
I had no poster presentations	Have one first-author poster on my CV by next time I apply	Run ideas by Dr. Who in May, run stats in June, submit to the International Neuropsychological Society (INS) in August, create poster by January, and present in February

the following year. This will keep you from scrambling in the months before you apply for internship, realizing that it is too late to obtain the kinds of experiences you need to be competitive. Here are some tips that we have for you:

- **Tip 1: Set a time in your schedule every week to track your clinical hours, assessments, and reports.** Don't leave this until the last minute. Make this a part of your weekly routine and devote 15 to 30 minutes to this task. There are some paid programs (e.g., Time2track) that you can use—remember to look up promo codes each year or check to see if your program offers a discount so you're not paying full price. You can also create your own excel spreadsheet—make sure you are tracking basic demographic data for your clients/patients, the specific tests in the battery for that assessment, the number of hours spent in face-to-face work (e.g., diagnostic interview; time spent testing, and feedback, even if you are observing), supervision (specify whether group vs. individual), and other hours (e.g., report writing). Also, track the number of neuropsychological reports you wrote that week.

- **Tip 2: Update your CV at least once every year.** Pro tip: It's even better if you get into the habit of updating it as soon as you complete something CV-worthy. Your poster got accepted to a local conference? Great! Add that to your CV. Oral presentation at a local conference? Started a new practicum? Won a travel award? Gave a talk to your community about the brain and aging? Taught a class? Submitted a grant? Gave a case presentation in rounds? Completed a 3-day neuroimaging course? Add these to your CV right away, and be detailed about what you did and the skills you gained. You can always cut back later if the details are unnecessary. Your future self will thank you.

- **Tip 3: Before the start of every year, review these numbers and compare them to your benchmarks.** Are you making good progress toward these benchmarks? In the categories where you aren't making as much progress, be intentional about how you want to use this next year to get closer to your end goal. If you don't have any research products in neuropsychology related topics, and your primary research is not related to neuropsychology, you will have to become creative. You could try contacting a neuropsychology practicum supervisor to see if they are working on a research project and offer your assistance with creating a database and analyzing data. You could also consider writing a review paper on a neuropsychology-related topic. How about your clinical work? Are you getting good-quality neuropsychology experiences (see Chapter 4 for what would constitute a good-quality experience)? If there are none available, you might have to forge your own way. Many trainees have come to us with success stories of how they cold-contacted a neuropsychologist in their community or a nearby academic institution, created a practicum experience, and ended up establishing a practicum site for graduate students in their program. On the flip side, if you realize that you have met or exceeded these benchmarks, give yourself permission to pull back a little and focus your efforts on the other areas that will help you become a competitive applicant for internship, like your milestones.

- **Tip 4: Review guidelines.** If your program does not require you to do this already, we would recommend reviewing the guidelines for practicum training in clinical neuropsychology—specifically, the exit criteria for practicum training. Be critical and honest about your abilities as you review where you are. If you have concerns about any of these areas, consider bringing this up with your supervisor and ask them whether you can focus more time in these areas. If you don't have the required coursework available through your program for neuropsychology specialization, supplement your knowledge. Chapter 11 of *The Neuropsychologist's Roadmap* provides a list of resources to assist with functional neuroanatomy, including textbooks, formal coursework, and free resources available on the web. There has also been a concerted effort in the field to increase access and availability of educational lectures; the KnowNeuropsychology Didactic

Series and NavNeuro podcasts are just a few ways to freely access educational content from neuropsychologists to trainees.

- **Tip 5: Be on the lookout for opportunities to network.** Neuropsychology is a relatively small field, so we understand that this is especially challenging if your mentor is not a neuropsychologist. One great strategy is to attend neuropsychology conferences. Ahead of the conference, email the conference organizers to see if there are any volunteering opportunities available (sometimes this comes with free registration). While at the conference, attend social events, talks, and poster presentations, and try to chat up the presenters when you can. Outside of conferences, you can network by joining a national, regional, or state organization. The National Academy of Neuropsychology has an online listing of organizations you can check out (http://tinyurl.com/4267yk6x), and many of these offer valuable opportunities for trainees to connect with peers/other professionals, opportunities for leadership and volunteering, financial support, and mentorship programs.

4

Preparing for and Obtaining a Predoctoral Internship in Neuropsychology

 Before working through activities on this topic, be sure to read through Chapter 2 of *The Neuropsychologist's Roadmap.*

This chapter is all about predoctoral internship (or "internship" for short). As with other chapters, we provide some practical advice for your application for and success at internship that is infused with feedback from 32 actual training directors/codirectors and supervisors who responded to items related to internship on our survey. We present these data throughout the chapter to help you better understand what they are looking for in internship applicants.

APPLYING TO INTERNSHIP

Like graduate school, applying to internship involves multiple steps over time, as well as several components that make up the application itself. In this section, we break down and review the application timeline and each of the required application materials.

The Application Timeline

See Table 2.2 in *The Neuropsychologist's Roadmap* (Block, 2021, pp. 37–38) for a suggested timeline of the application process, which starts with you assessing your readiness for internship long before applications are due. We've also provided a visual counterpart in Figure 4.1 here. Pace yourself! There are a lot of steps involved and a lot of moving pieces. Break up the process into smaller pieces, create (and stick to) your deadlines for each of those steps, and start

https://doi.org/10.1037/0000448-004
The Neuropsychologist's Workbook: A Hands-On Roadmap to Training and Developing Your Career, by C. Block and S. Hickle

FIGURE 4.1. Internship Application and Interview Timeline

	Spring					Summer			Fall/Winter			
	Jan	Feb	Mar	Apr	May	Jun	Jul	Aug	Sep	Oct	Nov	Dec
Assess readiness to apply			▓	▓	▓							
Consider fit factors					▓							
Create initial site list						▓	▓	▓				
Note application requirements						▓						
Update CV						▓						
Draft essays						▓						
Draft cover letter						▓						
Select final writing samples (if needed)								▓				
Finalize program list								▓	▓			
Solicit feedback on drafts								▓				
Request letters of rec								▓				
Draft edits									▓	▓		
Order/send transcripts										▓		
Finalize application										▓		
Submit application											▓	
Schedule interviews											▓	▓
Attend interviews (and do one just for practice)	█	█										█
Submit rankings		█										

Legend: ▓ = Fall/Winter of internship year
█ = Winter/Spring of internship year

Note. CV = curriculum vitae.

early so you aren't overwhelmed when November rolls around and applications are due.

Assess Readiness for Internship

Use the months of March through May to assess whether you are ready to apply for internship the next year. Exhibit 2.1 from *The Neuropsychologist's Roadmap* (p. 38) will help you in this assessment. We want to highlight factors that faculty members in graduate school training identified in our survey that would limit your readiness to internship. One consistent response was milestone progress, particularly dissertation progress. Not being far enough along on your dissertation can be a significant concern to internship programs because most students are too busy on internship to complete a dissertation. At a minimum, you should already have your dissertation proposed by the time you apply. If you are proposing an original research study, ideally you will already have your data collected by the time you apply or have a realistic plan to collect all your data before you start your internship (end of June or July).

A second factor limiting applicant readiness is if you don't have relevant and diverse clinical experiences. This applies to your referral types, clinical populations seen, diversity in your supervisors, as well as a breadth of clinical practicum experiences. On internship, trainees generally need to have a diverse background of experiences so they can readily adapt to new clinical rotations. A rotation might only be 3 or 4 months long, and trainees don't have the luxury of taking a full month to get up to speed. You want to demonstrate that you can adapt quickly to new types of clinical settings or populations based on your past experiences. Although it may not necessarily be a requirement to have had exposure to a particular clinical setting or population, such as a rehabilitation program or persons with traumatic brain injury, programs do like applicants who come in with some level of experience.

A lack of integrated neuropsychological report writing experience is also a crucial factor that would limit your readiness. As an intern, you will be expected to complete multiple neuropsychological reports per week, with a fast turnaround time. Being proficient and efficient with your report writing is essential, and the best way to develop this competency is by acquiring experience by the sheer volume of reports you've completed, getting critical feedback on them, and revising when necessary.

We recommend you set up a meeting with your mentor, dissertation advisor, and/or department chair to decide collaboratively whether you are ready for internship. Don't be discouraged if they say they don't think you are ready. Use that time with your mentors to get a good understanding of what steps you need to take, what skills you need to develop, or what experiences you need to pursue to become ready for internship.

Meeting the Minimum Benchmarks

We know it helps trainees to understand exactly how many clinical hours to strive for and how many reports are "enough" to be a competitive applicant. Survey respondents involved with internship training were asked about the number of hours and reports they would recommend trainees have before they are ready to apply to a predoctoral internship in neuropsychology. As you can see in Table 4.1, the range is substantial, and the answer will really vary based on who you ask. We've also included the information from a recent survey by Hirst et al. (2022), where neuropsychologists were asked what the minimum and average number of hours and reports were for a competitive applicant. Don't stress over specific numbers if you don't quite hit the average number of

TABLE 4.1. Survey Results: Minimum Clinical Benchmarks From Our Survey and Hirst et al. (2022)

Variable	Our survey results				Hirst et al. (2022) results		
	M ± SD	Median	Minimum	Maximum	M ± SD	Minimum	Maximum
Number of therapy hours	306 ± 132	300	75	500	405 ± 240	0	1,000
Number of neuropsychological assessment hours	410 ± 254	375	50	1,000	312 ± 313	0	2,000
Number of other assessment hours (achievement, psychodiagnostic)	167 ± 147	100	50	500	—	—	—
Number of supervision hours	310 ± 518	200	0	2,000	—	—	—
Number of integrated neuropsychological reports	—	—	—	—	29.8 ± 22.3	2	100
Number of adult/geriatric reports	32 ± 23	25	1	120	—	—	—
Number of pediatric reports	17 ± 13	20	1	40	—	—	—

Note. Data from Hirst et al. (2022).

hours in each category. Our recommendation is to focus on having good quality assessment practica (varied referral questions, diverse clinical populations, diverse experiences) and writing lots of reports. You can emphasize the quality of your experiences in your cover letter, curriculum vitae (CV), and essays. Also, once you've hit the average number of recommended hours and reports, focus on your milestone progress and your dissertation! Having 100, 200, or even 300 more hours than the recommended average isn't going to set you apart from your peers, especially if those hours aren't translating to more varied and diverse experiences. Defending your dissertation before you apply or go on your interviews will set you apart.

Consider Fit Factors

The purpose of the internship year is to complete training in the general practice of professional psychology. A critical but secondary goal is to further one's specialization in neuropsychology. This is an important distinction. Because internship is one of the last opportunities for you to get generalist training, a sizeable portion of the year will involve rotations that are not in neuropsychology. As you start considering the type of internship program that's right for you, you will want to identify other goals you want to accomplish during internship training—for example, in which clinical populations or psychiatric diagnoses do you want more training? Do you want your training internship to focus on assessment or intervention, or do you want a balance of both? Use the prompts presented in Exhibit 4.1 to brainstorm and shape the specific goals you have for internship training, which will help guide you as you look for internship programs.

Now, remember the fit factors that you identified and ranked for yourself when you were preparing to apply for graduate schools? You'll be using those again. Review the fit factors to consider in Exhibit 4.2, and use the worksheet from Chapter 3 (Table 3.2) to work through and weigh the options that are most important for you. Ask your mentors, supervisors, and current neuropsychology interns/postdoctoral fellows what factors were important to them when they were deciding to choose between programs. Try inputting some of your own fit factors and use it as you review internship programs. You may also find that as you go through the application and interview process, you identify additional fit factors you had not thought of before.

We also note that internship usually offers a combination of clinical training, research, and didactics, and there will be some variability across programs as to the exact weight of these factors, but in general, internship is considered a highly clinical year. It is not uncommon to have internships with no protected research time or any research obligations. You'll want to consider exactly how much research you will want to engage in at the internship level.

Do Your Homework

In Chapter 2 of *The Neuropsychologist's Roadmap*, take a look at Table 2.3 (p. 44) which provides several concrete ways for you to look up internship programs

EXHIBIT 4.1

Prompts to Help You Brainstorm Goals for Internship

Which skills, activities, or clinical populations do my supervisor(s) say are areas of training weakness/need?

In which types of approaches do I want to get more assessment training (e.g., fixed-flexible, Boston process)?

In which types of settings do I want to get more assessment training (e.g., inpatient, outpatient)?

In which clinical populations and diagnoses do I want to get more assessment training (e.g., stroke)?

With which age groups do I want more assessment training (e.g., pediatric, adult, geriatric, lifespan)?

In which types of approaches do I want to get more intervention training (e.g., cognitive behavior therapy, cognitive rehab)?

In which level of acuity do I want more intervention training (e.g., inpatient, outpatient)?

In which type of setting do I want more intervention training (e.g., Veterans Affairs, private practice, hospital)?

In which clinical populations and diagnoses do I want more intervention training (e.g., neurological)?

With which age groups do I want more intervention training (e.g., pediatric, adult, geriatric, lifespan)?

What do I want my training on internship to focus on (e.g., assessment, intervention, or a balance of both)?

Which types of referral questions have I not seen enough of (e.g., capacity, return to work, forensic)?

What types of mentorship/supervision have worked well for me, and what do I need more of (e.g., Socratic)?

Which aspects of diversity (e.g., cultural, ability/disability) could I benefit from getting more of?

Am I interested in conducting research on internship, and if so, in what area?

Are there any research skills that I want to learn/practice more (e.g., neuroimaging, structural equations)?

From what other learning experiences would I benefit (e.g., internship didactics, brain cutting rounds)?

Am I interested in seeking out leadership opportunities, and would I need mentorship in that?

Is it important to me to train under neuropsychologists who are board certified?

---

that provide training in neuropsychology. As with graduate school programs, we recommend that you write out your thoughts and observations as you review program websites and brochures to help you clarify quickly which programs are indeed a potential fit. It will also help you begin to sketch out the information that becomes important in crafting your training goals at a given program. Use the blank worksheet in Table 4.2 to help you keep track of and organize important information.

Because so many trainees apply to Veterans Affairs (VA) programs, we think it's important for you to know that you must meet all eligibility requirements to train at VA facilities. For instance, you must be a U.S. citizen. Also,

EXHIBIT 4.2

Fit Factors to Consider

Geographic location
Cost of living
Stipend
Program prestige and reputation
Work–life balance
Percentage of dedicated time to research
Research fit
Number of available supervisors who are board certified in neuropsychology
Supervision style
Clinical populations
Guaranteed first-choice rotations
Availability of professional mentors
Number of available neuropsychology rotations
Opportunities available for minor rotations of interest
Availability of postdoctoral fellowship program in neuropsychology at the same site or city

male applicants between the ages of 18 and 26 must sign a preappointment Certification Statement for Selective Service Registration before they can be processed into a training program. Transgender and gender-diverse applicants should note that if you were assigned male at birth and updated your documents to a different gender marker, you are still required to register. Individuals assigned female at birth and who updated their documents to male are not required to register (but some agencies may ask you to provide a Status Information Letter from the Selective Service indicating if you were or were not required to register—for more information, go to this website: https://www.sss.gov/register/who-needs-to-register/#p7). All information about eligibility requirements at the VA can be found on their website (https://www.va.gov/oaa/hpt-eligibility.asp). There is a checklist you can download to ensure you meet all eligibility requirements.

As you review internship program websites and materials, fill out the table, devoting one row to each program. At this stage, you are just gathering information and learning about what different programs have to offer and whether they could potentially be a good fit for you, so cast a broad net. We'd recommend putting anywhere from 15 to 20 programs on your list, with the understanding that this will be whittled down as you work through potential fit. Here are more specific instructions for how to fill out the table; we've added columns for you based on what we think are some factors that set programs apart and are important for you to consider.

- **Accreditation by the American Psychological Association (APA) and/or Canadian Psychological Association (CPA):** Indicate whether the program is APA- or CPA-accredited (whichever is most relevant to you), not accredited, or awaiting accreditation.

TABLE 4.2. Program Review Worksheet (Blank)

Program name	APA or CPA accredited	SCN member or NP emphasis	General program information	Program-specific information	Clinical training	Research training	Other

Note. APA = American Psychological Association; CPA = Canadian Psychological Association; NP = Neuropsychology; SCN = Society of Clinical Neuropsychology.

- **Society of Clinical Neuropsychology (SCN) member/major area of study:** Write down whether the program is listed in the training directory of the SCN and/or whether clinical neuropsychology is offered as a major area of study, an emphasis, experience, or exposure.

- **General program information:** Here, you can list information such as the program location (city, state/province), yearly stipend, and benefits. Benefits include options for health insurance and policies around paid time off, professional development (e.g., time off for conferences, interviews), sick days, and holidays. It could also include funding for travel to conferences or Examination for Professional Practice in Psychology study materials.

- **Program-specific information:** Here, list information such as the cohort size (i.e., number of general and neuropsychology interns being taken the next year) as well as the number of faculty in the program who are neuropsychologists (especially board-certified ones).

- **Clinical training:** Take notes on the structure/duration of the major rotations, type of clinics/clinical populations, any specialized training opportunities, and settings of interest. Include the other rotations available at the program (focus on the ones that are interesting to you), duration, frequency, and setting of the clinical minor rotation. Include information on typical assessment and therapy caseload, if that is available in the program's materials.

- **Research training:** Review the list of supervisors and their research interests, emphasizing the ones where you have matching research interests. Brochures will usually have a blurb for each supervisor that details their research interests. Note whether there is protected research time (yes/no), and if so, the number of hours per week

- **Other:** Here, you can make note of anything else that may be relevant to you. This could include making note of mandatory and optional case conferences, grand rounds (i.e., for medical departments such as neurology, neurosurgery, psychiatry, geriatric medicine), seminars, journal club, brain cuttings (i.e., a type of medical rounds in which a neuropathologist will dissect brains of recently deceased individuals to confirm/disconfirm a diagnosis or identify other previously undiagnosed brain disease/injury), or other professional development opportunities (e.g., opportunities for board certification–style fact findings). Be sure to include important information such as the application due date/time and interview notification dates.

Essential Elements of Your Application

Chapter 2 in *The Neuropsychologist's Roadmap* provides helpful tips for the essential elements of your application (i.e., cover letter, CV, four essays, letters of recommendation, possibly a writing sample). Pay attention to and keep track of important requirements for your application because some programs will want specific information included in the cover letter. For example, a specific paragraph on your research interests/projects, a paragraph on diversity, to whom you should direct your cover letter, or the code number for their program. Some will go as far as to indicate how this information should be formatted (e.g., headings, bullet points, bolded text). Use Table 4.3 after you narrow down your program list to keep yourself organized and to ensure that you follow all instructions when preparing your materials.

Letters of Recommendation

Most programs will ask for three letters of recommendation. Just like your letters for your application to grad school, your recommendation letters should be able to speak to your academic, research, clinical, and interpersonal dimensions. As a whole, your reviewers should be able to glean a picture of your academic, clinical (neuropsychology and general), research, and interpersonal skills. When you have decided on your letter writers, give them at least 1 month advance notice to author the letter. We highly recommend that you prepare a packet they can reference during this letter writing process. In this packet, consider including some or all of the following items:

- **Program list.** For each program, include the full program name (with department, if applicable), the name and credentials of the program training director, instructions on to whom the letter should be sent (and by what means), and clear due dates for the letters. Submission instructions will be simple—their letter will be submitted to the portal. You can use the same form from Chapter 3 (Table 3.7). Speaking as busy supervisors and letter writers ourselves, we can say with certainty: Reminders are very appreciated!

- **Shared experience list.** We also recommend including a bullet-point list (briefly) outlining experiences you've shared with that specific person. Did they teach one or more of your classes? If so, which, and what was your grade? Were you a teaching assistant for them? Did you publish or present anything together? If so, what and where? Did you work together clinically? If so, which rotations and populations?

- **Curriculum vitae.** You should also include an updated version of your CV.

- **Cover letter.** It may be helpful to include a sample cover letter from your application because this should include clear goals for your future that your letter writer may wish to reference. If you don't have a draft yet, at a minimum, you'll want to provide a bulleted list of specific goals that you have for internship. Your letters are another opportunity for the people reviewing your application to determine whether you are a good fit for their program, and an easy way to do that is for your letter writers also to include information about your goals for internship and career.

It's appropriate to provide reminders at the 1-week mark, assuming that the letter itself has not been written yet. In the reminder, include the due date and information on who the letter will be going to (i.e., program/training director name and email, or weblink if relevant).

TABLE 4.3. Application Requirements for Internship Programs

Program name	Deadline	Name of training director	Program address	Match ID	Cover letter requirements	Requires writing sample?	Other

Update Your Curriculum Vitae

The same advice that we provided regarding your CV in Chapter 3 still stands. Keep your CV visually streamlined and consistent, well structured, and with only the most relevant content to allow application reviewers to locate the information they need quickly to decide on whether to extend an interview offer.

We want to draw your attention to the "Clinical Training" section in the CV template we provided in Chapter 3 (see Exhibit 3.2). Internship is primarily a clinical year, and thus you'll want to highlight important information about your neuropsychology practica. In this sample, you can see that all the supervisors you worked with and their credentials/board-certification statuses are included. Also, be specific about the training activities that took place (e.g., were you involved in test administration, scoring, diagnostic interviewing, report writing, feedback?) and the specific neurological, medical, and psychiatric diagnoses you gained exposure to while on that rotation. If you have a lot of clinical rotations during your training, consider breaking them up into two separate sections, one for all your assessment practica and another for all your therapy practica.

We also advise that you don't go overboard on fancy fonts: Keep bolding, italicizing, and underlining to a minimum. That way, when you do use some flourish, it becomes much more effective in highlighting the most special parts of your CV. For example, look at the research portion of the sample CV in Figure 3.3 from Chapter 3. Notice that the trainee's name is underlined in any paper/poster presentations or publications that are listed. It draws the eye, doesn't it? Clearly number all presentations and publications so it's easier for your application reviewer. If you have many kinds of publications, it's permissible to separate these into subsections (e.g., peer-reviewed publications vs. non–peer-reviewed).

Cover Letter

The cover letter is a crucial part of your application to help your program identify whether you are a good fit. We've provided a sample cover letter (Exhibit 4.3), as well as a list of helpful do's and don'ts provided by neuropsychologists who regularly review applications to internship programs (Table 4.4). Overwhelmingly, the advice given was that the cover letter should explicitly address the fit between the program and your own goals. Take the time to read through the program materials and use this information to personalize the letter, and express genuine interest and enthusiasm for the program. One other piece of advice provided was that if you have only had experience with attention-deficit/hyperactivity disorder or autism from graduate school, address whether you want to remain in that vein or not. People reviewing your application understand that sometimes these are the only opportunities trainees have for assessment and will want you to address explicitly in your materials whether you want to remain in that area of assessment or branch out. To help you avoid some of the items from the "don'ts" column, we've created a checklist (see Exhibit 4.4) for you to complete for each program to ensure that you aren't making avoidable mistakes.

EXHIBIT 4.3

Sample Cover Letter

October 30, 20XX

Training Director Name
Address

Dear Dr. XX and Selection Committee Members:

I am writing to express my interest in the XX internship training program, specifically the **Neuropsychology** rotation. Based on my review of your program materials and conversations with students who have completed their internship and training at your site, I believe your site offers a training experience that aligns with my career goals of becoming a board-certified neuropsychologist in a medical center. My graduate studies at XX doctoral program, as well as my clinical experiences at external practicum sites, have laid a foundation of clinical skills in assessment and intervention settings within a scientist–practitioner framework. I am eager to obtain a well-rounded internship training experience that will allow me to expand on these skills and develop new competencies.

I have identified multiple aspects of your internship program that are in line with my training goals. My career goal is to practice in a medical center, and I would like to increase my exposure to a variety of medical and neurological conditions, hone my diagnostic interviewing skills, and increase my proficiency in providing feedback to patients and their families. Your site offers multiple neuropsychology rotations that target this goal, such as the Neuropsychology Outpatient Service, Geriatrics Clinic, and Inpatient services. These rotations would provide opportunities to conduct evaluations for patients with a variety of conditions while concurrently learning about the neurobiological mechanisms that underlie the behavioral presentations of common and rare conditions within an evidence-based framework. I am particularly interested in gaining more experience working with older adults with various types of dementia through the Geriatrics clinic. In addition, my training so far has been exclusively in outpatient settings, and I am eager to gain assessment experience in an inpatient setting. I was excited to see that there are numerous opportunities to gain exposure to patients in acute stages of injury through several clinics.

Another feature of your program that interests me is the opportunity to lead a cognitive rehabilitation and psychoeducational group for patients with neurological and medical conditions. One of my training goals is to become proficient in administering evidence-based interventions to improve daily functioning in individuals who have cognitive impairments. I was able to explore this interest briefly through an external practicum that involved providing treatment for young adults with neurological conditions to improve adaptive functioning skills; I am eager to obtain specialized training that will target this goal and to extend my experience by working with adults.

Another aspect of your site that I find appealing is the opportunity to gain rehabilitation psychology experience through the Rehabilitation Psychology rotation. My first clinical experience was in a Polytrauma/TBI clinic at a VA. There, I received exposure to patients with medical and psychiatric comorbidities (veterans who had sustained TBIs but also suffered from trauma, mood disorders, sleep disturbances, pain, and fatigue). In that setting, I had several opportunities to observe neuropsychologists work in an interdisciplinary team with other medical professionals and use the results of the assessments to identify a personalized plan for each patient. I could see how treatments

(continues)

EXHIBIT 4.3

Sample Cover Letter (*Continued*)

were most effective when there was a conceptualization that considered the complex interplay of mood, cognition, and health for each patient and identified ways to adjust their treatment based on potential personal and/or environmental barriers to treatment. Since that time, my goal has been to be able to engage directly in team discussions and planning and provide tailored, evidence-based interventions. I believe that my effectiveness as a health care provider will be enhanced by gaining experience working in interdisciplinary teams to assist with the rehabilitation of patients whose mood, cognition, and health interact in complex ways.

I also value the resources and training that your site provides through supervision and didactic activities that complement clinical work. I believe that receiving supervision from board-certified neuropsychologists will allow me to learn from individuals who have specialized competences and will help further my own goal of being board certified. I am also excited about opportunities to attend the Neuropsychology Seminar Series, Neuroimaging Lecture Series, Neurobehavioral rounds, and Epilepsy Case Conferences to learn from a wide range of in-house and community experts. I have been fortunate to receive didactic training on brain–behavior relationships and case conceptualization through my graduate program and external practica, and I am eager to continue developing proficiency in these areas.

Finally, I am interested in the research opportunities available at your site. During graduate school, I collected and analyzed neuropsychological and neuroimaging data for a study investigating outcomes in adults who had acquired brain injuries when they were children. I am currently preparing my dissertation defense. Alongside practicing as a clinical neuropsychologist, my long-term career goals include conducting research in clinical populations by using neuroimaging techniques to explore the neurobiological underpinnings of behavior and cognition. There are numerous research labs at your site that align with my interests, such as the Core Neuroimaging Center, the Geriatric Laboratory, and the Memory Disorders Research Group. Your site has incredible resources to support students interested in neuroimaging research, and I am enthusiastic about any opportunity to become involved in any of these research labs during internship.

In sum, I believe that the internship training site at the XX is a setting where I could extend my training and develop new skills. The breadth and depth of training experiences available at your site are remarkable and fulfill many of my training goals. I also strongly adhere to the scientist-practitioner model and wish to train at a site that embodies this philosophy through both clinical and research domains. I appreciate your consideration of my application and welcome the opportunity to meet with your faculty and current interns. I look forward to hearing from you and learning more about the exciting opportunities that you offer.

Sincerely,

XXXX, MA

TABLE 4.4. Cover Letter Do's and Don'ts

Do	Don't
✓ Clearly define your goals for internship and highlight your strengths.	✗ Restate everything on your curriculum vitae (e.g., list all your prior practica placements) or on the program website.
✓ Demonstrate the fit between your short- and long-term goals and that specific program.	✗ Submit a cover letter with the wrong program name.
✓ Clearly articulate what your short- and long-term goals are and how you believe that specific program will help you meet them.	✗ Copy and paste the list of internship experiences from the program website without any synthesis of how this fits with your personal goals.
✓ Write clearly and concisely.	✗ Express interest in opportunities not available at that program.
✓ Take the time to find and include the training director's names (including the codirector).	✗ Overemphasize research goals; internship is mostly a clinical training endeavor.
✓ Highlight information that is not obvious in other parts of the application.	✗ Submit an overly generic letter.
✓ Include the names of specific individuals with whom you would want to work.	✗ Submit a letter with significant spelling and grammatical errors.
✓ Include the names of specific rotations that you think will meet the goals you've provided.	✗ Submit a letter that goes beyond two pages.
	✗ Name drop.

EXHIBIT 4.4

Cover Letter Checklist

Task

☐ Date is in the top left corner

☐ Training director's name in the top left corner and spelled accurately

☐ Program name and address in the top left corner

☐ Correct Match ID for track

☐ Program name and spelling are correct throughout the letter

☐ Rotation name and spelling are correct throughout the letter and accurately described

☐ Faculty names are accurately spelled throughout the letter

☐ Didactics names and spelling are correct throughout the letter and accurately described

☐ Formatting follows any requirements on the program website/brochure

☐ Includes all requested content from the program website/brochure

☐ Final copy edits: check for typos and grammatical errors

Essays

We want to impart some additional advice we received from neuropsychologists who review internship applications when we asked them, "What are you looking for in the essays? For example, what makes a strong essay? How personal should the essays get? What are your 'red flags' in an essay?" Overall, there was a consensus that strong essays first and foremost reflect solid basic writing skills. As one neuropsychologist wrote,

> [I'm] looking for the quality of the writing more than anything: clear, concise writing. They should be clear, well-written, and grammatically correct. Poor writing conventions stand out to me because our profession, either clinical or research, requires a ton of professional writing.

Spend time looking at the syntax, scour your essays for typos, and ask for help making your writing concise if you struggle with this. The number one red flag mentioned by the people taking our survey related to writing mechanics (e.g., typos, grammatical errors, lack of clarity/flow).

Second, essays should be genuine and let your personality shine through. One survey respondent wrote, "I like to learn something about the person that I can't get from their CV in the autobiographical essay." The essays should provide more information about the person as an individual, versus a rehash of a CV. Many of the people we surveyed cautioned against sharing very personal or controversial details in the essays, noting that this is an area in which an individual can harm their application by oversharing. One respondent wrote, "Do not tell me you got into psychology because of your own mental health conditions. Although that might be true . . . you have very little space to tell a rounded story about your journey." We know this is a fine line, but in general the essays should be personal enough so the reader gets to know the applicant but formal enough to remain professional. Stay away from controversial topics, and only disclose personal information that would be considered appropriate in professional settings. As the saying goes, "Be yourself—but be your best self."

On the other hand, don't spend too much time trying to achieve the perfect essay because, frankly, such a thing doesn't exist. One survey respondent wrote,

> It is rare that an essay really blows me away, and I can't think of a single time when an essay was a key factor in who received a higher rank (unless the essay was very poor). I've had many students get so caught up in writing the perfect essay they lose sight of how important it is to simply convey your experiences, goals, and passion for neuropsychology. Make sure your writing mechanics are on point and that you have good organization for all essays, but don't stress too much about finding that perfect hook or anecdote.

To summarize, ideally you'll want to aim to write a unique essay, but don't worry too much if you don't have one. Focus more on the quality of your writing. Put more effort into avoiding overly personal details that could serve as a red flag.

We also recommend using case examples in your essays where they are relevant. They are concrete examples that provide helpful information about your theoretical information, clinical skills, approach to diversity, and respect for your patients. One common red flag that was cited related to narcissism and arrogance regarding the scope of your abilities or influence. One survey respondent noted: "Be mindful that you are still a trainee. We are looking for examples that are appropriate to your level of experience. I want to hear about good boundaries, professionalism, theory-informed intervention, and guidance from supervisors when appropriate." Following are some other tips that we want to pass along regarding your essays: (a) Explicitly state your dissertation progress and anticipated defense timeline in your research essay; (b) if you identify with a historically marginalized population, explicitly state this in your cover letter and personal essay; (c) your diversity essay should indicate self-reflection of your own status, humility, and willingness to learn; (d) and finally, some neuropsychologists admitted that there were certain topics they've seen a lot of: enjoying puzzles, saying you are interested in neuropsychology because of a family member who had dementia, and saying you love the brain and want to study the brain because it's so interesting.

Writing Samples

Writing samples aren't always required, but chances are at least one of your programs will request one. We asked survey respondents to rank the factors that were most important to them when reviewing reports. There was a clear consensus: Writing quality was in everybody's top three factors. Conceptualization was in the top three for 94% of our sample. About half of respondents indicated that submitting a report with a neurological population was in their top three. The length of the report and the complexity of the case were the two least important factors, so we recommend you do not use these factors to pick your sample report.

Overall, we recommend picking a straightforward case with a neurological diagnosis that highlights your strong writing and conceptualization skills. We additionally recommend you avoid diagnoses that have some controversy in our field (e.g., nonverbal learning disability, chronic traumatic encephalopathy). This is to avoid the possibility that someone reviewing your report will disagree with the content of your report and make negative conclusions about your application. And this almost goes without saying, but make sure any writing samples that are reports or clinical notes are fully deidentified to standards outlined by the U.S. Department of Health and Human Services (2024). Also be sure to have your supervisor review and approve.

Finalizing Your Program List

September and October are good months to finalize the list of graduate programs to which you intend to apply. Use the fit factors worksheet you completed to help you finalize your list, prioritizing the programs that have higher totals. How many programs should be on your final list? On average, we would recommend somewhere between 10 and 15 programs. You may feel tempted to add more programs if you are feeling anxious about your prospects. Applying to more programs isn't necessarily better, especially if you can't demonstrate that you are a good fit. As you read the program materials, if you are unable to pinpoint why it is you want to apply or have a hard time personalizing your cover letter, chances are the people reviewing your application will feel the same way even if you may be more than qualified.

Making Yourself Competitive

We wanted to share some of the survey responses from neuropsychologists who review applications for internship (see Figure 4.2). We asked them to choose (up to) 10 factors that are most important to them when reviewing an application to a graduate program, and we've tallied up their responses based on the percentage of people in our survey who considered that factor one of their top 10. As you can see, and consistent with what we've been saying all along, almost everyone considered the fit between the applicant's stated goals and what the program can offer as one of the top 10 factors for almost everyone surveyed. Other clear factors that are considered the most important: the quality of your cover letter (60% rated this factor as one of their top 10), the strength of your recommendation letters (80%), the number of assessment reports (70%), and the number of neuropsychology externships/practica completed (73%).

We also want to highlight the factors that were not selected as the top 10 most important in an application. Involvement in leadership, grant writing/funding experience, number of oral presentations or posters at academic conferences, and graduate school cumulative GPA were not rated as the top 10 most important factors. We are not saying that these experiences are worthless or undesired. But we provide these numbers to help inform you as to which factors are broadly considered the most important by neuropsychologists reviewing applications.

We often get questions about research productivity and how many publications, oral presentations, and/or posters would be expected of a competitive applicant. The data from our sample of neuropsychologists are provided in Table 4.5, combined with the results from another research survey (Hirst et al., 2022) that broke down the number of publications into first authored versus coauthored publications. To be a competitive applicant, we recommend trying to publish at least two manuscripts (and in at least one of them you should be the first author). Try to submit one poster every year to a neuropsychology conference. This is not to say that you won't match to an internship if you don't have these numbers, but these are good benchmarks to strive for if you want to be a competitive applicant. It does become increasingly crucial for you to have research experience specific to neuropsychology; we specifically asked neuropsychologists how they would view it if an applicant had posters, presentations, and/or publications but none of them were related to neuropsychology, neuroscience, or neurology topics. Only 25% indicated that they would view this experience as positive, 40% viewed this experience as negative, and 33%

FIGURE 4.2. Survey Results: Most Important Factors When Reviewing an Application

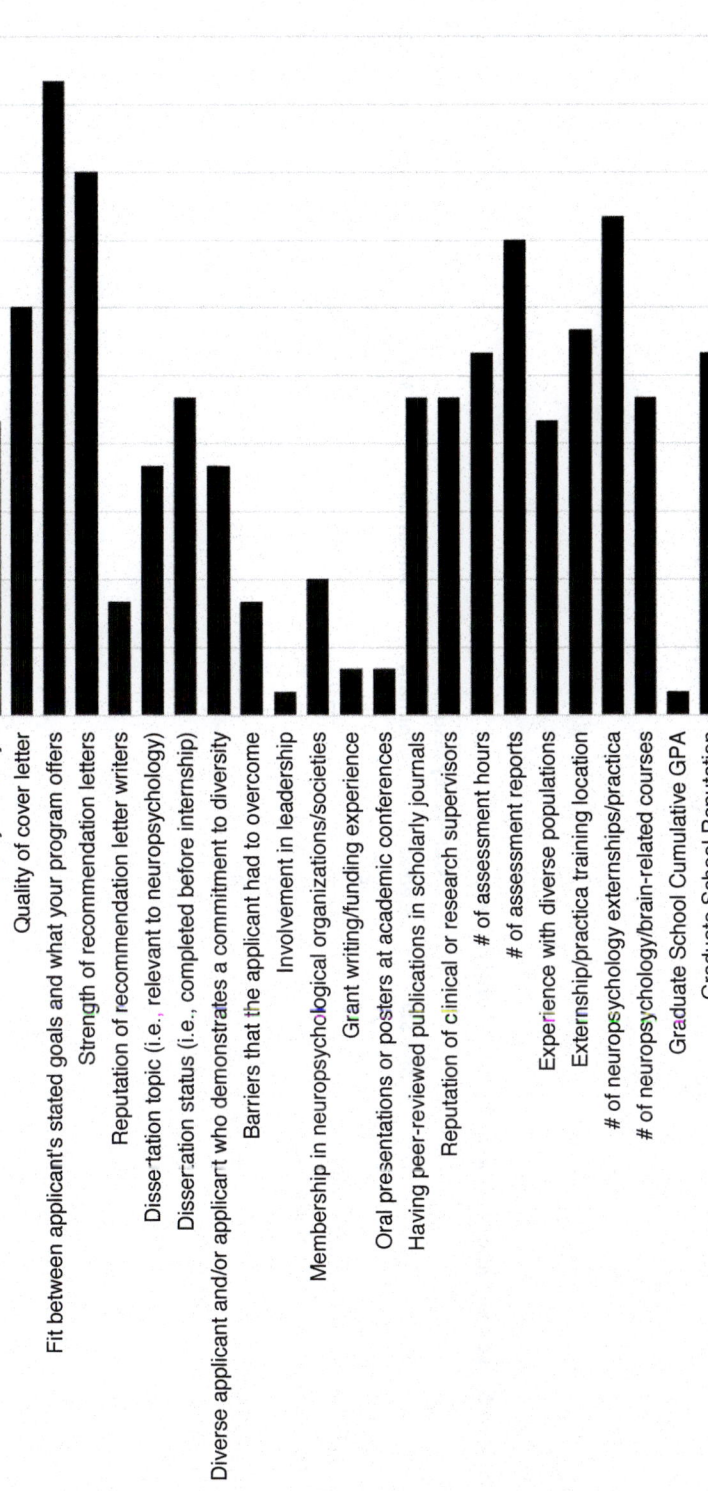

TABLE 4.5. Survey Results: Minimum Research Benchmarks

Variable	Our survey results				Hirst et al. (2022) results		
	M ± *SD*	Median	Minimum	Maximum	*M* ± *SD*	Minimum	Maximum
Number of publications	2.0 ± 1.3	2	0	5	—	—	—
Number of first-author publications	—	—	—	—	1.5 ± 1.4	—	—
Number of coauthor publications	—	—	—	—	2.5 ± 1.8	—	—
Number of oral presentations	1.5 ± 1.6	1	0	5	2.0 ± 1.9	—	—
Number of posters	4.4 ± 3.1	4	0	15	4.1 ± 2.9	—	—

Note. Data from Hirst et al. (2022).

were neutral. If your primary research lab in graduate school is not in a neuro-psychology-, neuroscience-, or neurology-related discipline, consider working with one of your neuropsychology practicum supervisors to publish at least one poster.

Scheduling Interviews

After you have submitted your applications, you'll have roughly 2 to 3 weeks before emails start rolling into your inbox saying that you've been invited for an interview. Most programs will offer several interview dates and ask you to reply indicating which dates you would prefer. You'll want to answer this email as quickly as possible so you can maximize the chance that you get your first choice. When we say as quickly as possible, we literally mean within the first 5 to 15 minutes. Keep the volume up on your devices and turn on notifications for emails so you'll know the moment the emails come in. In our experience, we've found that Fridays in January tend to be popular interview dates offered by programs. If programs offer dates that aren't Fridays in January, try to select those interview dates as your first choice.

Another tip we have for you is to create a spreadsheet right after you submit your applications that has all your programs and their scheduled interview dates (usually they will be in the program materials). If they have not provided updated interview dates, you can still make an educated guess by looking at the interview dates they offered the year before. When you have all the information in one place, it will be easier to identify your first choice for the interview date for each program. See if there are any interview dates for one program that don't overlap at all with any other programs—that is usually a good first choice because there is no chance you'll have to choose between two programs. Then look at the programs that offer the fewest inter-view dates. You'll want to select your first choice interview date for those programs because they will have the least flexibility compared with programs that offer more dates. Continue going through all the programs so you have a first choice for interview date each. Keep this information handy (e.g., print it out and put it in your wallet) so you can easily access this information when you get an email notification offering an interview. That way you can quickly reply to that email with your first choice for interview date.

If you haven't heard from any programs by the middle of December with an interview offer, it's time for you to reflect. Be honest as you answer the questions in the readiness self-reflection exercise in Table 4.6. If you struggle with being objective, ask a trusted mentor or fellow graduate student to read through your materials and help you answer these questions. If you answered "no" to any of the items in the application section, revise your materials so that the answer becomes a clear yes before submitting your application to any additional programs. If you've found more than a few answers in the "no" column in the candidate readiness section, it's time for you to consider whether an internship with a neuropsychology focus is feasible for you. Know that board certification in neuropsychology is possible without having

TABLE 4.6. Readiness Self-Reflection Exercise

Application	Yes	No
Did my letter-writers write a strong letter of support?	☐	☐
Do my goals match what the site offers?	☐	☐
Did I express my goals for internship and how the site is able to meet these goals in my cover letter?	☐	☐
Did I personalize my application materials (i.e., did I mention specific rotations, supervisors, and research opportunities available at the site)?	☐	☐
Are my essays/cover letter well written and free of spelling and grammatical mistakes?	☐	☐
Do I make it clear which clinical populations I've worked with, and how much neuropsychology-specific experiences I've had so far in my materials?	☐	☐
Are my materials free of "red flags" (e.g., inappropriate levels of self-disclosure, arrogance regarding the scope of my abilities and my influence in a patient's or client's care)?	☐	☐
Applicant	**Yes**	**No**
Do I have enough face-to-face hours?	☐	☐
Do I have good-quality neuropsychology practica experience?	☐	☐
Do I have experience writing full reports?	☐	☐
Have I written at least 25 full reports?	☐	☐
Have I worked with neurological populations (e.g., dementia, traumatic brain injury, stroke)?	☐	☐
Can I realistically complete my dissertation before the end of internship?	☐	☐

any internship experience in neuropsychology. However, a 2-year doctoral fellowship is required. It will be hard for you to be competitive for a post-doctoral fellowship if you don't have the requisite neuropsychology experience in graduate school or internship.

We know that often it is not financially or personally feasible to wait another year to apply for internship. One option would be to consider applying for programs where neuropsychology is offered as a minor rotation, or an adjunct experience, so you can still get some exposure to neuropsychological assessment. There are also other rotations where you can get exposure to the patient populations that could work as a "bridge" to a postdoctoral fellowship, such as an internship with an inpatient rehabilitation emphasis or geriatric psychology. If dissertation progress might be the primary concern from the program's perspective, consider adding more details to your application materials to emphasize your detailed plan for how you will finish as much of the dissertation as possible before starting internship. If you decide instead that you want to focus on getting good-quality neuropsychology experience and defend your dissertation in the next year so you can be competitive for a strong internship with an emphasis in neuropsychology next year, there is absolutely no shame in that either. You have a great head start on all your application materials for the next year.

Interviewing at Internship Programs

If you have received one or more offers for an interview, congratulations! Many applicants see the interviews as daunting. We challenge you to frame your perception. By reading this chapter, you're already increasing your odds of matching. And interviews can actually be fun. Do you enjoy conferences, where you meet new people and hear about the cool things they're doing? Well, interviews are not all that different.

Interviewing for internship is not all that different from interviewing for graduate school. The same tips we provided in Chapter 3 (e.g., thinking about the fit between your goals and the program, being professional) still apply. Here is the advice that survey respondents (who are actively or at some point have been involved in reviewing applications and interviewing at the internship stage) have for you. We'll update these tips with internship-relevant information.

- **Tip 1: Think about the fit.** Be prepared to talk about the fit between your goals and what the program has to offer. We recommend that you review the program materials before the interview so you know what the program offers, and the faculty members there. If you took our advice from earlier in this chapter and personalized your cover letters, this should be easy. At this point, you'll have a stronger sense of your career goals than you did for graduate school, and you should be able to articulate how that internship program fits in with those goals. Fit can also be demonstrated by talking about specific gaps in your training, and how the program can round out your training experience and set you up for postdoctoral fellowship. The more detailed you can be when talking about that program's rotations, clinical populations offered, didactic opportunities, and supervisors and how each of these components can help you in your training journey and meet your goals, the better.

- **Tip 2: Prepare and practice.** You will prepare by doing your homework on the program and the supervisor(s), preparing questions to ask, and preparing answers to some common questions in advance so you can be polished and specific in the interview. Practice with a mentor, other faculty in your program, a program supervisor, or even a faculty member you do not know. They can give you tips on how you present and if you seem overly anxious or overly confident. Take their advice seriously and ask for suggestions on how to address any concerns. Here are some additional things to prepare:

  ✓ **Prepare a 1-minute introduction of yourself.** This should include mention of your strengths (the things you're good at), skills you have obtained, in what ways you would like to grow on internship, and how the specific program can help you do that. Make sure to maintain a humble tone when you talk about your skills so you don't come across as overly confident or arrogant.

  ✓ **Prepare a 1-minute explanation of your dissertation.** This should include a very brief background, your main hypotheses, main findings (or anticipated findings), and where you plan on taking this line of research next (e.g., publication, presentation, future studies). Difficulty describing your dissertation could be seen as an indicator that you struggle to communicate complex material; make sure to practice with your mentor so they can give you feedback on the clarity of your communication.

✓ **Prepare several case examples—specifically, assessment cases.** Include a concise overview of the referral question, presenting concerns, background history, summary of testing data, conceptualization, and relevant recommendations. Find an example of a case that went well and a case that did not go well. For the latter, be able to talk about what you learned from this case. Make it a point to talk about how you sought out supervision appropriately. You'll also want to talk about the elements of diversity that were relevant to the case (e.g., did it affect normative data selection? Test selection? Your conceptualization? Your recommendations?).

✓ **Prepare to talk about an ethical dilemma.** What was the situation that happened, and what specifically was ethically concerning about it? To wow your interviewer, try to tie the ethical issue to the principles and standards outlined in the American Psychological Association (2017) Ethics Code (see https://www.apa.org/ethics/code). Many interviewees get caught up in trying to pick something overly complex because they want a dilemma with a wow factor, but we encourage you to keep it straightforward. What are some everyday ethical issues that arise? This could include things like recordkeeping, informed consent, access to interpreter services, and using the appropriate test norms. If you're not sure, run your planned ethical dilemma by a supervisor or two to ensure it's appropriate.

✓ **Prepare to talk about one good and one challenging experience you have encountered in supervision.** For the first, what was good about it? What did that mean to you then, and going forward? For the second, what was challenging about it? And how did you handle it? Be sure to select an example where you handled that experience professionally. Again, if you're not sure, then run it by a supervisor or two to ensure it's appropriate.

✓ **Prepare your own questions.** Make sure to have questions for every interviewer, because it shows your interest and (hopefully genuine) enthusiasm for the program. Try to avoid questions that are already in the program materials, website, or brochure; instead aim for ones that are higher level and show you're thinking critically about the program and its potential fit. It may help for you to write out a list of questions you want to ask, including some that would be handy to pull from if there is a lull in the conversation (see Exhibit 4.5 for some sample questions). Try to keep at least two or three subjective questions in your back pocket that you can use more than once; it's totally fine to ask the same question to multiple interviewers (it even helps you get different perspectives).

EXHIBIT 4.5

Sample Interview Questions

Sample Questions for and About the Program

- What is the best part about this site? What is the most challenging?
- What are the strengths of the program? Weaknesses?
- What is the professional climate at your institution? Do you interface often (and well) with other specialties?
- How does this program balance the broad and general training in clinical psychology with specialty training in clinical neuropsychology?
- How is rotation order decided in this program?
- Can you walk me through your rotation structure and what a typical day looks like?
- What are the most common referral sources, referral questions, and patient populations for neuropsychological assessment on this rotation?
- When it comes to neuropsychological report writing, can you tell me about the typical length and structure of your reports?
- Do neuropsychological report expectations (i.e., length, structure, turnaround time) differ between supervisors?
- What research opportunities are available? Can you give me some examples of what current or prior trainees have done in your program in terms of research?
- What kinds of opportunities are available for multidisciplinary work or consultation?
- Are there other didactic opportunities outside the program? Are trainees allowed to attend?
- Are there opportunities for trainees to provide supervision? Are there other didactic or experiential opportunities for supervision?
- What is your supervision style?
- How do you foster trainee clinical skills from a developmental perspective?
- How does your program contribute to a trainee's preparation for board certification?
- What does the program do to support diverse students and/or students from nontraditional backgrounds?
- What postdoctoral experiences are available at this site?

Questions You Should Be Prepared to Answer

- Tell me a little bit about yourself.
- Tell me why you wish to be a neuropsychologist.
- Why us? What about this site in particular interests you and would make you good a fit?
- What are your personal strengths and weaknesses?
- How will this program help you round out your training?
- What types of clinical populations do you want to work with?
- Tell me about a therapy case you had. How did you conceptualize the case, what approach did you use, and what was the outcome?
- Tell me about an interesting neuropsychological assessment case you had. What was the presenting concern, how did you approach the battery and testing, and what were the results and impressions?

(continues)

EXHIBIT 4.5

Sample Interview Questions (*Continued*)

- Here are some sample neuropsychological test data for patient Harry Potter. I am going to give you a few minutes to look it over. Talk me through the results, what they mean, and the differential diagnosis.

- Tell me about your dissertation. How is it progressing, and what are your expected findings?

- What are your research interests and how have they evolved? Where do you see your research going in the future?

- What sort of supervisors have you had? What type of supervision works best for you and why? What type of supervision do you find challenging and why?

- What are you looking for in a supervisor?

- Describe an ethical dilemma you've had, how you tried to resolve it, and how the situation turned out.

- What are your future goals? Where do you see yourself in 5 years? (*Note:* Try to say more than wanting to be a board-certified neuropsychologist in an X setting. Be specific.)

One question we recommend being thoughtful about: What makes a successful trainee in your program? Some interviewers argue that this question is of dubious value because, in a sense, it could be the same personal and professional qualities at any program: having sensitivity to ethical and cultural issues, respect for others and building/maintaining good working relationships, timeliness, being conscientious, an openness to learning, and a willingness to be challenged. If you opt to ask this, be judicious about which programs, interviewers, and current trainees you ask. Interviews can go faster than you think, and we think the questions you ask should be ones yielding the most valuable information specific to that individual program. Never tell an interviewer you have no more questions; this is considered a red flag by some interviewers.

- **Tip 3: Relax and reframe.** It's natural to feel anxious about interviews, but try to reframe that. Maybe your anxiety is excitement at this wonderful new step in your training journey, one that you've been working hard toward for years. And if you've gotten the interview offer, the program already believes you are competitive (doesn't that feel good to know?). At the point of interview, it's really all about demonstrating fit and letting your personality shine. In a sense, that makes interviews seem less daunting. To be frank, some neuropsychologists even weigh the interview less during the ranking process because they are so subjective; the interview is truly an opportunity for them to see if the applicant will have their goals met at the program, seems genuinely interested in what they have to offer, and doesn't seem to have a completely poor "fit" with the culture of the program. And as we mentioned earlier, interviews can be fun! Many trainees have shared with us their surprise at how much they enjoyed interviewing and how collegial the process was for them. Many make life-long friends along the way. That's the norm, not the exception.

- **Tip 4: Wear comfortable clothing.** We recommend business casual attire at the very least. That means some combination of a dress shirt or blouse, slacks or skirt, or coat and tie. You want to be remembered for your professionalism (including professional appearance). We recommend choosing clothing that's professional but comfortable. Interview days can sometimes be long and tiring. This is especially important for shoes, doubly so if you're attending an in-person interview. Tours are often a part of the interview process, and your feet won't be happy after walking around large, sprawling medical centers in shoes that are stiff, too small, or have tall heels. When it comes to virtual or telephone interviews, we still recommend you dress the part; interviewees reported that it does help them feel more mentally prepared and polished.

- **Tip 5: Take extra time for setup if you have a telephone or video interview.** More and more interviews are moving to telephone and video conference formats, which has been great for the field because trainees no longer have to endure the significant stress and cost that winter travel posed. The day before, prepare and test your home setup. Make sure you use a computer or laptop rather than tablet or smartphone. Run a quick test of your internet speed to ensure reliable and high-quality signal, and we recommend using a free checker such as SpeedTest (https://www.speedtest.net). Many web-based platforms such as Zoom or Teams require a minimum download speed of 1.5 Mbps and upload speed of 2 to 4 Mbps (depending on whether it's a single or group call/meeting). On SpeedTest, you can check download and upload speeds of your connection by viewing the numbers next to the teal downward arrow (download speed) and purple upward arrow (upload speed). Now that you've ensured your internet signal, do a quick test to make sure your speakers (and headphones or microphones, if you're using them) are working optimally. And do a quick practice run with someone you trust. They can help you catch if there's anything distracting in your environment (e.g., too many visible objects or extraneous noise), and we recommend interviewing in a private setting with a relatively clean environment. Some artwork, books, or plants are fine—but there is a fine line between this and clutter. A practice run can also help catch when you're exhibiting any distracting habits (e.g., poor lighting, sitting too close or too far from the camera). We want to emphasize that you be extra mindful of nonverbal habits. Virtual interviews lose a bit of the liveliness of in-person interactions, thus body language becomes even more important. Easy ways to indicate interest and engagement include sitting up straight and leaning forward slightly, nodding as people talk, using good eye contact, smiling, and making hand gestures. Avoid crossing your arms, touching your face, playing with your hair, sighing, or fidgeting. Also, try not to touch your phone or look off screen, as this can be misinterpreted as disinterest or even as reading material off screen (your interviewer can tell where your eyes are looking, and it's obvious when you are reading from a written script).

- **Tip 6: Be professional.** Remember your manners because first impressions count. First, be on time. Be kind and respectful to everyone you see, including any staff, trainees, or other applicants. Overconfidence and arrogance toward other applicants were considered a red flag for the neuropsychologists that we surveyed. Don't speak ill of any past mentor, supervisor, colleague, or peers. Try to refrain from using slang or too many fillers such as "um," "uh," "like," and "you know." Also refrain from cursing, which might seem like it goes without saying—but believe it or not, it does happen! It's okay to exhibit a sense of humor, just make sure it's appropriate to the situation. Finally, make sure your mobile phone ringer is turned off.

- **Tip 7: Take notes.** Have a notepad with you during your interviews. It's not only okay to jot down some quick notes, but we recommend it. And once the interview day is finished, we recommend that you write down important information and impressions about the program as quickly as you can. This includes things that may not have been in the program materials, any surprises you encountered, how current interns seemed (tired? happy? disgruntled?), and the general impression you came away with (like you met your perfect match, or did you find yourself trying to fit a square peg in a round hole?). Your notes become a very helpful reference when you are ranking programs. It doesn't have to be organized, and it doesn't have to be pretty. But having a written account of answers to your questions and your impressions will ensure that you have a more accurate recall of that program when ranking.

- **Tip 8: Send thank you emails but do pay attention to when programs ask that you don't send them.** Writing thank you emails is certainly not a requirement, but it can be nice to do especially if you are genuinely interested in the program. If you choose to write a thank you email, keep your communication brief and professional. And again, please make every note of the programs that explicitly tell you not to send thank you emails.

In looking at the results from our survey, the factors that respondents considered most and least important when interviewing applicants are included in Exhibit 4.6. On the basis of what you've read so far, is it any surprise to you that clinical fit and personality fit were considered the most important factors when interviewing applicants? We will note that demonstrating research fit/ promise was one of the least important factors when interviewing applicants for the people who took our survey ranked factors. However, we add the caveat that for sites that have a heavy research component or internship sites that have options for interns to stay an additional year for a research fellowship, research fit during the internship application may be more crucial.

EXHIBIT 4.6

Survey Results: Ranked Interview Factors

Top-Ranked Factors (Most Important First)

Demonstrates personality fit with faculty, supervisors, and other trainees
Demonstrates clinical fit/promise
Being well-prepared for the interview (e.g., high-quality questions/responses to interview
  questions)

Bottom-Ranked Factors (Least Important First)

Nonverbal behaviors/mannerisms
Demonstrates research fit/promise
Quality of responses to standardized interview questions
Quality of general verbal interaction

RANKING INTERNSHIP PROGRAMS

We recommend checking out page 51 of *The Neuropsychologist's Roadmap*, which provides overall guidance on the ranking process. Use the fit factors you created for each program. Don't discount factors such as the "feel" you got from the program. If you have additional questions, reach out to the interns or supervisors there for answers!

It is possible that you may feel stuck between two fit factors. For instance, one program may be perfect in terms of clinical fit, but geographically is in the last place on earth you would ever want to live. There really is no right answer to how to rank in this scenario. Consider your own personal values to help you decide what is truly important to you and make choices that align with your values, which will help ensure that you find meaning and satisfaction in what you do. Take a look at the values quiz we've developed, which you can use to help guide you while making ranking decisions (see Table 4.7). The values listed in the table all relate to different aspects of work and invite you to think about how important that value is to you. Be honest with yourself—there are no right or wrong answers.

When you've finished, look at the values that are "very important to me." Keep these values if you feel stuck when deciding. If your number one value is to have your workplace be in a location that is geographically convenient to you and this trumps all other values, then give yourself permission to rank based on geography. Thinking about your values can help you "weight" different fit factors. A couple of things to keep in mind: Internship is 1 year, and you still have postdoctoral fellowship to get more experience to specialized neuropsychology training. If there are training experiences and clinical populations that are not offered in a specific internship program, there will be additional training opportunities available to you, so don't feel you are shutting the door because of your selection.

TABLE 4.7. Values Quiz for Ranking Decisions

Value	Not important to me	Somewhat important to me	Very important to me
Taking risks			
Achievement			
Solving problems			
Helping others			
Teamwork			
Autonomy (e.g., working well with mentors that are hands-off)			
Working alone (e.g., working well independently/solo)			
Working cooperatively (e.g., working well with other trainees, staff, providers, researchers)			
Working flexibility (i.e., according to my own schedule)			
Being supervised by multiple people			
Being supervised by one person			
Being able to supervise others			
High/frequent communication with others			
Low/infrequent communication with others			
High/frequent movement during the day			
Low/infrequent movement during the day			
Prestige/reputation of program			
Financial reward/high earnings			
Career progression			
Being valued/recognized			
Receiving feedback that is constructive/critical			
Receiving feedback that is affirming/positive			
A competitive and demanding environment			
A warm and nurturing environment			
A fast-paced environment			
A slower paced environment			
Being innovative			
Detailed work/precision			
Learning/growth (i.e., an opportunity to expand my skills and knowledge)			
Predictability/stability			
Change, adventure, and variety			
Diversity, equity, and inclusion			
Work–life integration/balance			
Having fun at work			
Geographic location			
Other:			
Other:			
Other:			

Note. Once you are finished checking all items, highlight or place a star next to the ones you marked as "very important." Write these out on a separate sheet of paper, and let them guide some of the questions you ask during interviews as well as the considerations you have when jotting down postinterview notes.

What to Do If You Don't Match

If you are left without a program match in Phase I, know there is always a Phase II round in which programs that also did not match have openings. We can say with confidence that we've seen many excellent programs have openings in Phase II! If you happen not to match in the first round, meet with one or more supervisors/mentors to come up with a plan to submit for the second round. If you still don't match, we recommend reviewing the tips in Chapter 2 of *The Neuropsychologist's Roadmap*, as well as reviewing the strengths and weaknesses in your application (ideally with a mentor) to come up with an action plan to make you a stronger applicant for the next year. Make your goals SMART—specific, measurable, achievable, relevant, and time-bound (see p. 303 of *The Neuropsychologist's Roadmap*). Set a timeline for yourself, with clear, actionable goals that you can track. And good luck!

5

Preparing for and Obtaining a Postdoctoral Fellowship in Neuropsychology

 **Before working through activities on this topic, be sure to read through Chapter 3 of _The Neuropsychologist's Roadmap._**

This chapter is all about postdoctoral fellowship ("fellowship" for short). We provide some practical advice that is infused with feedback from 36 actual training directors/codirectors and supervisors who responded to items related to postdoctoral fellowship. We present data from this survey throughout to help you better understand what these individuals are looking for in fellowship applicants.

APPLYING TO POSTDOCTORAL FELLOWSHIP

Like graduate school and internship, applying to postdoctoral fellowship involves multiple steps over time, as well as several components that make up the application itself. In this section, we break down and review the application timeline and each of the required application materials.

The Application Timeline

As noted in Chapter 3 of _The Neuropsychologist's Roadmap_ (Block, 2021), a postdoctoral fellowship involves 2 years of intensive and specialized training in neuropsychology. Most fellowships entail a combination of clinical training, research, and didactics. Some fellowships are nearly entirely (or entirely) research-focused, and this is something as an applicant that you will have to decide when weighing your personal "fit factors."

https://doi.org/10.1037/0000448-005
The Neuropsychologist's Workbook: A Hands-On Roadmap to Training and Developing Your Career, by C. Block and S. Hickle

It may be hard to believe, but the period for considering these fit factors begins right as you start your internship. For a timeline of fellowship application, interview, and ranking/matching, please refer to Figure 5.1 in this book as well as Table 3.1 in *The Neuropsychologist's Roadmap*. Your internship year will go by quickly, and during that period, you'll be busy applying, interviewing, and securing a fellowship so you want to be able to have enough time to think about what you really want and need. Some internships begin as early as June, but most begin in July or August, so we think those make good months to start assessing your strengths and weaknesses. You may also wish to consider your ultimate career trajectory. Are you aiming for a more clinical career? And is that one without any research or one that blends the two? Would that be a career focusing on neuropsychological assessment, rehabilitation, or a blend of the two? Or are you instead aiming to pursue an academic career in a university department? We recommend you review Chapters 6 through 8 in *The Neuropsychologist's Roadmap*, which do a good job of overviewing your potential career options. Coming up with a tentative answer to this question can help guide whether you seek a research or clinical fellowship.

Consider Fit Factors

July and August are also good months to start sketching out what sort of fit factors are important to you. Use the worksheet from Chapter 3 (Table 3.2) to work through and weigh the options that are most important for you. As an example, in Table 5.1, you can see our prospective fellowship applicant highly values programs that are located in the mid-Atlantic region, are in the match, offer training opportunities across a range of institutional settings, have both neuropsychology and rehabilitation experiences available, and have more than one board-certified neuropsychologist that can serve as supervisors. You may also wish to think about financial considerations here: If a program is at a

FIGURE 5.1. Fellowship Application and Interview Timeline

Steps during internship year	Spring				Summer				Fall/Winter			
	Jan	Feb	Mar	Apr	May	Jun	Jul	Aug	Sep	Oct	Nov	Dec
Considering fit factors								■				
Looking for sites	■								■	■	■	
Submitting applications	■									■	■	
Interviewing	■	■										■
Rankings/Match		■										

Legend: ■ = Fall/Winter of internship year
        ■ = Winter/Spring of internship year

TABLE 5.1. Fit Factors (Sample)

Fit factor category	Item and response			Score weights
Program factors	Match vs. nonmatch status	X	1	Program in match
			0	Program not in match
	Program type/ setting		3	Academic medical center or affiliated Veterans Affairs (VA)
		X	2	Consortium program
			1	Nonacademic affiliated VA or private hospital
			0	Other
	Program supervisor(s)	X	2	More than one board-certified supervisor
			1	One board-certified supervisor
			0	No board-certified supervisors
Individual factors	Geographic location		4	Mid-Atlantic
			3	South/Southeast
			2	Midwest or Southwest
		X	1	West Coast or Northeast
			0	Other
	Interest match		1	Has neuropsych and rehab rotations
		X	0	Has neuropsych rotations only
	Total			6 points

qualifying institution for the federal Public Service Loan Forgiveness program, then any payments you make during fellowship count toward the required number of payments (you can check an institution's availability online at the Federal Student Aid, Department of Education website: https://studentaid.gov/pslf/employer-search). Try inputting some of your own fit factors and running it through a few fellowship programs.

As you're considering these fit factors, from your internship start date through September and October make sure you get plenty of face-to-face time with your internship supervisor(s). One or more will potentially be authoring a letter of recommendation for you, and you want them to know you well enough to write a strong letter. Set up weekly supervision or mentoring sessions and come prepared with questions or ideas for discussion. If you need some ideas on potential topics for discussion (and helpful tips), refer to Figure 17.1 in *The Neuropsychologist's Roadmap*.

LOCATING POSTDOCTORAL FELLOWSHIP PROGRAMS

September and October are good months to begin crafting and finalizing the list of fellowship programs to which you intend to apply. How many programs should you apply to? In our survey, respondents felt that applicants should apply to no less than six and no more than 12 programs (on average), although the ranges for each of these values was much wider—with the lowest number of programs ranging from one to 13 and the highest number of programs ranging from five to 20. All in all, we think you are safe applying to somewhere between eight to 10 programs. There are several ways to locate programs. One is through word of mouth, and you can rely on your growing network of peers and supervisors/mentors for this. Another is to look at online repositories, including the list of member programs in the Association for Postdoctoral Programs in Clinical Neuropsychology (APPCN; https://appcn. org/member-programs), the training directory sponsored by the Society for Clinical Neuropsychology (SCN; https://scn40.org/training-directory/), and the jobs listing through the International Neuropsychological Society (INS; https://www.the-ins.org/job-postings). X/Twitter is also growing in popularity as a place where research-focused postdoctoral positions may be announced.

It is certainly helpful to monitor all relevant neuropsychology listservs, as many fellowship (clinical and research) positions are advertised through them. Some suggestions include the listserv sponsored by the SCN's Association of Neuropsychology Students and Trainees (see https://scn40.org), the American Academy of Clinical Neuropsychology's community discussion or pediatric sub-specialty special interest group lists (https://theaacn.org/discussion-forums), and the NPSYCH listserv (https://neurolist.com/index.php?option=com_content& view=article&id=86&Itemid=335). As we noted in previous chapters, if you use Microsoft Outlook, you can set up an alert to be notified any time you get an email containing the word "fellowship" or "postdoctoral" in the subject line. See Chapter 3 for steps to accomplish this.

As these programs are advertised, you will need some way of sorting through them to determine whether they are a potential fit. Put your thoughts to paper. We find that it is helpful to consider a given program based on a few key factors. Allow us to direct your attention to Table 5.2, which contains a worksheet you can use to complete your review of a program with these factors in mind. Here is some information to help you understand what goes in each column:

- Program name: This is self-explanatory, folks.

- What fits: This refers to experiences and activities that already match what a program offers, such as (but not limited to) the program's training model (e.g., scientist-practitioner or clinical scientist), major clinical populations served, acuity of clinical services (i.e., inpatient or outpatient), or research productivity and content. These demonstrate that you already have some foundational knowledge and/or experiences to prepare you adequately for the rigors of a particular program. You could also pull information from the fit factors form you completed for that program.

- What's new: This refers to experiences and activities a program offers that you as an applicant do not have yet, or maybe have less of. These should be in line with your stated training goals. Things to consider would be similar to the "what fits" column, including training model, clinical populations served, acuity of clinical services, or research productivity and content.

TABLE 5.2. Fellowship Program Review Worksheet (Blank)

Program name	What fits?	What's new?	Other	Faculty of interest

- Other: Remembering that your training is more than just clinical work and research, this would cover all other potential things involved in your fellowship such as opportunities for continued structured learning, activities designed to help prepare you for board certification, diversity/equity resources or opportunities, credentials of current faculty, potential for mentorship in professional development or leadership/advocacy, and more. Select what would be of importance to you as the applicant. Do you prefer a site that is heavy in didactics? What didactics? A weekly "fact-finding" series that could help you better prepare for board certification? Or maybe that this program allows its fellows to attend the medical school's neuroanatomy course? Is it important to you that X number of the faculty are board certified? What about them serving leadership roles in national/international organizations, which could be relevant if you wanted mentoring in leadership development or support in networking for research/professional opportunities or jobs? Personal factors are useful to include such as geographic location, salary, leave, or other benefits.

- Faculty of interest: It may be useful to also list faculty with whom you would be interested in working. You could also list their board-certification status, associated clinical rotations or populations of interest, research activities, or maybe even organizational affiliations.

APPLYING TO POSTDOCTORAL FELLOWSHIP PROGRAMS

As we get into the application and interview steps, it's a good time to pause and mention that the APPCN website has a helpful listing of frequently asked questions on the application, interview, and match/ranking process for fellowships (https://appcn.org/applicants-faq). September and October are good months to begin putting your application together. Update your CV, select and de-identify a few sample evaluation reports (and run them by a supervisor for review and approval), and make the request to your letter of recommendation writers. You will also need to author a cover letter for each individual program and likely will need to request transcripts. As in applying to all prior steps of your training journey, be sure to keep all materials well organized and clearly titled.

Update Your Curriculum Vitae

First, you will want to update your CV. In our survey, respondents were asked to rank—out of 25 possible items—the most and least important factors when reviewing fellowship applications. While "CV" wasn't a specific item in this question, in looking at Exhibit 5.1, you can see that the top five items are things that can be readily found in your CV—meaning that it is just as important to attend to your CV as it is other components of your application. In Chapter 3 of this workbook, you can find a sample CV template as well as some handy tips—and we recommend you revisit both (Exhibit 3.2 and Table 3.5).

EXHIBIT 5.1

Survey Results: Ranked Application Factors

Top-Ranked Factors (Most Important First)

Graduate school reputation
Internship reputation
Number of neuropsychology externships/practica
Externship/practica/internship training locations[a]
Diverse applicant and/or applicant who demonstrates a commitment to diversity

Bottom-Ranked Factors (Least Important First)

Quality of sample neuropsychological reports
Quality of cover letter

Note. [a]Academic medical center, private hospital, community hospital, Veterans Affairs medical center, children's hospital, rehabilitation hospital, private practice, and so on.

At the fellowship level, you may consider adding a few additional sections based on your experience, including any grants or other research funding that you may have been awarded ("Research Funding"), mentored/ad hoc journal review experience ("Journal Review Positions"), or teaching or research assistant experience ("Teaching Positions" and/or "Research Assistant Positions"). Depending on the nature of the program you are applying to, you may wish to shift sections around. For example, you can better highlight your research accomplishments by placing that section ahead of clinical training, professional affiliations/positions, teaching, and so on (or vice versa for more clinically oriented programs). It may be helpful to divide up your publications section into empirical/original articles versus those that are literature reviews or book chapters. If you've accrued quite a bit of clinical experience up until this point, it may be helpful to divide your rotations up into those that are general clinical and those that are neuropsychology specific. Remember: Keep everything straightforward and well organized so reviewers can quickly get the information they need when scanning your CV. As mentioned in the graduate school chapter, reviewers often spend less time than you think reviewing it. Make that time count!

De-Identified Sample Reports

Next, you will need deidentified sample reports. Not all programs require this as part of your application, but you want to be prepared in case any do. In our survey, the majority of respondents (88%) indicated that their fellowship program required sample neuropsychological reports as part of the application. These did not appear to be weighed heavily, however. When asked to rank the most and least important factors when reviewing fellowship applications, quality of sample reports were ranked last out of the 25 items presented in this specific survey item. However, they are still considered and do deserve some thoughtfulness from you. The majority of our respondents felt that a good demonstration of *brain–behavior conceptualization* was the most key aspect that they looked for in a sample report. Ranked in order from most to least important, this was followed by overall writing quality, the fact that the evaluation was performed on someone with a neurological condition, quality of the report recommendations, the test battery employed, case complexity, and report length. So keep these in mind when selecting your sample reports. You want to select one or more that demonstrate your range of exposure to different neurological populations, employment of accepted neuropsychological measures in a coherent battery, ability to integrate test findings with behavior observations and presenting history, and ability to communicate the diagnostic picture clearly as well as provide meaningful recommendations. You want to show off the knowledge and skills you've acquired in the years of training you've accumulated up until this point. Conversely, you would want to avoid submitting overly lengthy or brief reports that rely on minimal measures (or measures that are not well known or well standardized), on a patient with a nonneurologic condition, or that doesn't translate to report recommendations. Another red flag is when an applicant submits reports that are not fully de-identified to Health Insurance Portability and Accountability Act (HIPAA) standards. Review all sample reports at least once, with an eye to de-identification alone. Check your report against standards outlined by the U.S. Department of Health and Human Services (2024; https://bit.ly/3IFVSSI) and have your supervisor review and approve.

Letters of Recommendation

Finally, you will need letters of recommendation. Similar to other application steps, the majority of fellowship programs ask for three letters. Do not submit any more than the program requires, unless they specifically stipulate that this is permissible.

Who should be your letter writers? Ideally, you would have someone who knows you well from your doctoral program; this could be your primary advisor/ mentor or your dissertation chair. You would also want one or more advisors/ mentors from your internship program. If you only happen to have one available, it is fine to have someone else affiliated with your doctoral program write a letter. This could be someone who taught a course you excelled in, or someone who supervised a clinical rotation—the key here is to have someone who knows you well and can write you a strong letter. Since the original release of *The Neuropsychologist's Roadmap*, the survey of 88 postdoctoral fellowship programs released by Driskell et al. (2022) showed that 86% of respondents felt that recommendation letters written by neuropsychologists were either *essential* or *very important* (however, this dropped slightly to *very* or *somewhat important* when it came to letters from a board-certified neuropsychologist). We would add that if your choice of neuropsychologists is limited, then it is certainly permissible to have a nonneuropsychologist author the remaining letter; it is vastly better for you to have a strong letter from a nonneuropsychologist than a weak or mediocre letter from a neuropsychologist.

Similar to our advice in other chapters, give your writers plenty of time to author the letter. One month in advance should be sufficient, being mindful of other potential factors (e.g., if your letter writer will be out of town or it's the holiday season, maybe allow more time). Again, consider preparing a packet of information for your letter writers to reference as they go. For a listing of what information is helpful to include, see Chapter 3 of this workbook (Table 3.7). For fellowship programs, especially those that are research-focused, it may be helpful to include an abstract or brief description of your dissertation project (and its status). Much less common, but still optional and worth noting, would be copies of rotation evaluations from internship so your letter writers can reference your progress (and other glowing reviews you may have received). Be judicious in your inclusion of these optional materials, however, because you don't want to overwhelm your letter writers with too much extraneous information. And be sure to provide written reminders to your letter writers— along with the letter due date and information on the letter recipient (e.g., program director name and email, or web link if relevant).

Cover Letter

A cover letter is also part of every application. This is your chance at a first impression, so it deserves just as much attention as other parts of your application. In our survey, the general consensus of respondents was that a good cover letter should be no more than 1 to 1.5 pages in length, tailored to the aspects of the program that drew your interest, outline why you are a good fit for this program, and clearly articulate your career goals (including making a direct connection between these goals and how the program helps you to meet them). Use the information you gleaned from the program review activity we discussed earlier in this chapter (see Exhibit 5.1) and from the program's own brochure or website. We recommend the following structure to your cover letter:

- Paragraph 1: This paragraph should be an introduction to you and your intent. Provide your name and credentials, current training status, and graduate and internship institutions. You might also consider including your primary goal here. For most, that would entail becoming a board-certified clinical neuropsychologist in X setting (academic medical, Veterans Affairs [VA] health care, private practice, forensic, and so on). For more research-focused applicants, it may entail becoming a grant-funded, productive neuropsychologist in X setting (e.g., academic, academic medical, industry). Programs want to see that your ultimate goal aligns with what they offer.

- Paragraph 2: This paragraph should indicate what existing experiences you already have qualify you for a given program. Think broad: It could be the type of therapeutic orientation or intervention(s) offered by the program (e.g., cognitive-behavioral, cognitive rehabilitation), the type of assessment approach (e.g., process-oriented, fixed-flexible), age groups served, clinical populations served, research or administrative or supervision opportunities, and so on. Anything that shows you can "hit the ground running," so to speak. Programs typically want fellows that come prepared enough to be ready to take full advantage of what they offer, not ones who would require lots of remediation.

- Paragraph 3: Use this paragraph to detail what experiences you lack that the program offers and would help you achieve. As in Paragraph 2, think broad. Fellowship is about more than just neuropsychological assessment. Addressing other facets of the program shows that you are being thoughtful in your approach to the application and interview process as well as fellowship training itself.

As a final note for the cover letter, you can highlight some of your activities and accomplishments, but make sure this isn't something that could just as easily be obtained from a quick glance at your CV. Be sure to look over your letter with an eye toward any punctuation, grammatical, and syntactical errors. Have a supervisor or peer look it over to help ensure it is well organized, well written, and sufficiently formal in tone. In addition to your cover letter, many programs will likely ask for your graduate transcripts, so be prepared to request those in advance—and allow yourself plenty of time.

INTERVIEWING AT POSTDOCTORAL FELLOWSHIP PROGRAMS

Give your interview as much attention as your application. In the Driskell et al. (2022) study, the interview was identified as the second most important factor in ranking applicants—and this was across program settings (i.e., academic medical center, VA) and population (i.e., adult, pediatric, and lifespan). In years past, most interviews took place at the annual February meeting of the International Neuropsychological Society (INS)—and a few still do. This typically kicks off with an applicant breakfast on the Tuesday of the week of INS, followed by interviews that may occur throughout the remainder of the week. There is usually dedicated space for interviews in the conference hotel, but with so many going on, don't be surprised if they spill out into the lobby seating area or hotel restaurant. A smaller subsection of programs prefers to interview on site. And for a variety of equity, access, financial, technological, and other considerations, most programs have shifted to virtual interviews.

Now, interviews at this level of training might feel a little different. They might feel more like recruitment ("Here's why we want you to come here!") than evaluative ("Tell us why you want to come here") in nature. The exception to this may be VA medical centers, which require performance-based questions as part of the hiring process (because you will technically be an employee as well as a postdoctoral fellow); for a list of questions, see U.S. Department of Veterans Affairs (2018). Other things won't be all that different. You will still be asked about your educational background, clinical work, and research interests. You will still be asked "Why apply to our program?" You will still see a variety of interview styles—some warm and fuzzy, others more businesslike. You will likely interview with a current trainee or two. As in other levels of training, it is good to do a practice interview. This helps shake out the nerves but can also be helpful in practicing responses to some of the more common questions (for a listing of sample interview questions, please refer to Table 3.2 in *The Neuropsychologist's Roadmap*). We recommend one to two practice interviews with neuropsychology supervisors, and it can be especially helpful to do one with someone you might be less familiar with to better approximate the actual interview. Ask for feedback not just on the length, content, and clarity of your responses but also to identify any potentially distracting verbal or nonverbal mannerisms.

In our own survey, respondents were asked to rank what interview factors they found most important. As you can see in Exhibit 5.2, notice that clinical fit and personality fit were rated as the top two most important. Here are some comments from the neuropsychologists we surveyed; notice again that most of these comments related to goodness-of-fit:

- "Be honest! We already know you are qualified, so the interview is really about fit. Be honest about what you want so you end up somewhere that fits."

- "Manage anxiety. Be yourself. If you have an interview, you are a competitive candidate. The faculty are looking at you and wondering if you're a good interpersonal fit."

- "Know what you do well and communicate that clearly. Tell me what aspects of my program would help you achieve your goals."

- "Have plenty of questions—the quality of your questions says a lot about your preparation and how invested you are in learning about the site."

- "Be prepared for a lengthy process and know we are trying to get to know you and want you to get to know us to ensure a match between you and us."

EXHIBIT 5.2

Survey Results: Ranked Interview Factors

Top-Ranked Factors (Most Important First)

Demonstrates clinical fit/promise
Demonstrates personality fit with faculty, supervisors, and/or other trainees
Being well prepared for the interview (e.g., high-quality questions)
Quality of general verbal interaction
Demonstrates research fit/promise (tied with the next item)
Quality of responses to standardized interview questions (tied with the previous item)

Bottom-Ranked Factors (Least Important First)

Workplace-appropriate appearance and attire
Nonverbal behaviors/mannerisms

By doing the legwork on fit factors in advance, you will already be attuned to this well in advance of the interview—and, based on your engagement with the material in this chapter, should already have some material you can use in response to this question!

Making Yourself Competitive

To make yourself a competitive fellowship applicant, it's helpful to understand what programs are looking for. The Driskell et al. (2022) survey also provides some helpful information regarding clinical training. At both the graduate and intern levels, academic–medical and Veterans Affairs hospitals were ranked as the top two desired training sites. Following these, in order from most to least desired, were rehabilitation centers, private or community-based hospitals, university/college clinics, psychiatric/state hospitals, and private practice. Across any of these sites, respondents indicate that an average of 61.5% time engaged in clinical work was most ideal—with the minimum time spent being 40% (again, averaged across respondents).

In our survey, we asked these individuals to rank their top 10 most important factors when reviewing applications to their fellowship program, as well as rank their bottom five least important factors. The top two rated items were the reputation of your graduate program (#1) and reputation of your internship program (#2). If you did not attend a well-known or well-regarded program, do not fear. Also ranked highly were the number of neuropsychology externships/practica or internship rotations, their location, and an applicant who is diverse and/or demonstrates a commitment to diversity (refer back to Exhibit 5.1). Ranked toward the bottom were the quality of the sample neuropsychology reports and quality of the cover letter.

Although research productivity was not necessarily a top-ranked factor, we did ask respondents some specific questions regarding what exactly constitutes a "productive" applicant. In terms of the number of posters to be considered a competitive applicant, somewhere between three and five seemed to be the consensus of respondents from more clinically focused programs; in contrast, respondents from more research-focused programs generally considered somewhere between eight and 10 posters to be sufficient. When it came to oral presentations, the consensus of all program types was that one or two was sufficient. For publications, there was a clustering of responses that could not be easily differentiated by program type; the majority, however, responded with a range of 1 to 5 publications (39% reported that 1 to 2 publications would be considered competitive, while 44% felt 3 to 5 were sufficient). The relationship of research posters, presentations, and publications to neuropsychology, neuroscience, or neurology was highly desired; nearly half (47%) of respondents indicated that a lack of relation to these topics would be viewed negatively. In the Driskell et al. (2022) survey, an average of three peer-reviewed publications was expected of competitive applicants (2.8 ± 1.6), although the range was fairly wide, spanning anywhere from no publications to upward of 10. The highest value was among non-APPCN member fellowship programs (3.7 ± 1.5), likely because this category is more apt to include more research-focused fellowships. A similar pattern was observed for number of peer-reviewed presentations, which was an average of six overall (5.8 ± 2.7) and higher than that in non-APPCN member programs (6.6 ± 2.6).

So what does this all mean? In your training, try to accrue several neuropsychology externships/practica and internship rotations. It can be especially helpful if they are in academic–medical and VA settings, but ultimately any neuropsychology training in any setting is better than none. Consistent with the Houston Guidelines criteria (see the Houston Conference on Specialty Education and Training in Clinical Neuropsychology Statement Policy Statement at https://uh.edu/hns/hc.html), you want roughly half of your clinical training to be in neuropsychology. As far as research goes, even if aiming for a clinical career, you want to be able to demonstrate some level of scholarly activity in the form of posters, presentations, and publications—more so if you're aiming for a research-focused career. In your clinical work, research, and other administrative/professional activities, seek out experiences related to equity, diversity, and inclusion as a means to demonstrate your commitment to diversity.

Self-Reflection

It's important to take the time to reflect on what is most important, and most enjoyable, to you. What sort of fellowship experience are you looking for? Do you have any particular preferences about programs that are in the match versus not? Read on for more information.

Clinical Versus Research

One pressing question for many applicants is whether to commit to a clinically focused fellowship or a research-focused fellowship. A simple decision tree is included below (Figure 5.2). But know that the choice may not be so black and white! Many clinically focused fellowships do have faculty that are productive in the scholarly sense, allow some dedicated research time, and have research resources available (e.g., datasets, statistical consultants, funds for poster printing and conferences). If you want to be board certified, this may be more ideal because clinically focused fellowships will already afford you the necessary training and supervision hours to pass the credentials review portion of the board-certification process. But even in some research fellowships, you can still conduct some clinical work (or may be able to negotiate for some protected clinical time).

However, if your desired pathway is heavily dedicated to research and grantsmanship, then you may wish to consider a fellowship that is more research focused. This would likely be persons who wish to pursue a career in academic, academic–medical, or industry settings. There are some research positions available in VA medical center settings as well. Essentially, you want a fellowship that provides ample opportunities for training and mentorship in grant writing, data analysis, and manuscript preparation—particularly in areas

FIGURE 5.2. Decision Tree for Research Versus Clinical Fellowship

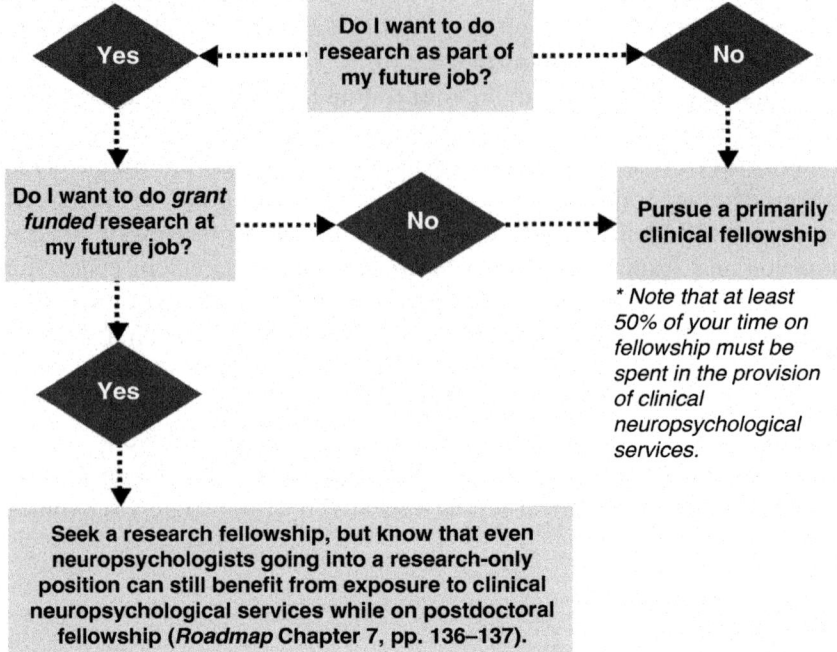

directly relevant to your career plan. For example, you would seek a research fellowship at a program specialized to Parkinson's disease if in the future you intend to pursue grant-funded research in the area of movement disorders; it wouldn't make much sense to spend a large portion of your fellowship training performing research in children with traumatic brain injury if what you ultimately intend to pursue is a research career in Alzheimer's disease.

Match Versus Nonmatch

Another question is whether to apply to match versus nonmatch programs. There are a variety of reasons why programs prefer to be match or nonmatch. These could include philosophy of training, equity/fairness in recruitment, and control over candidate selection. Ultimately, the decision of which to apply to comes down to you. Our advice? Seek to apply to programs that are the best fit for you, regardless of match status. If you do apply to match programs, just make sure you familiarize yourself with the rules of participation and, in particular, how to manage any preemptive offers from nonmatch programs appropriately (see the APPCN's Match Agreements page: http://natmatch.com/appcnmat/rules.html).

Success on Fellowship

Once you have secured your fellowship, congratulations! You'll have a little bit more time before you have to worry about the next cycle of interviews (for your first job). We will note that many training directors suggest taking the Examination for Professional Practice in Psychology (EPPP) during your fellowship year (see Chapter 6 in this workbook for more information), so you're not quite out of the woods in terms of having to take more exams. Aside from EPPP, we also encourage you to use this time to start thinking ahead to board certification. Be sure to track all hours throughout all of your fellowship. You can (and should) take advantage of the American Board of Professional Psychology's "early entry" option (https://abpp.org/application-information/application-types/early-entry-application) as a more affordable way to start banking credentials. We recommend that you remain mindful during fellowship as you think about your goals for your career. Imagine yourself at that ideal first job—what sorts of skills and experiences will you wish you had during fellowship when you had the luxury of having mentors at the ready? Make sure to advocate for yourself if you are not getting those skills and experiences! Fellowships can be flexible, and it is possible that your fellowship program may be able to be creative and provide these additional opportunities for you as you work toward your next step: the first job.

6

Professional Licensure and Credentialing

 Before working through activities on this topic, be sure to read through Chapters 4 and 16 of _The Neuropsychologist's Roadmap._

This chapter is all about getting licensed and credentialed. This is the step that occurs after graduation (although some steps of this process, like the Examination for Professional Practice in Psychology [EPPP], can be taken during graduate training) but before you can actually practice as a clinical neuropsychologist. Chapter 4 of _The Neuropsychologist's Roadmap_ (Block, 2021) delves into licensure in further detail than we'll do here, but this workbook can serve as a helpful study and organizational companion during the process.

LICENSURE

Licensure represents official recognition of your qualifications for professional practice. To be a practicing neuropsychologist in any clinical capacity, you must have an active license in professional psychology (outside of one or two states, there are no licenses for neuropsychology). Obtaining a license is a multistep process. You must (a) decide which state you wish to apply to; (b) apply and undergo a credentials review; (c) once approved, take the EPPP examination Parts 1 and 2; and then (d) take any remaining state-specific written and/or oral examinations. When it comes to deciding on which state, we find the Association of State and Provincial Psychology Board's (ASPPB) PsyBook to be a very handy resource for figuring out specific state requirements (see http://psybook.asppb.org). State psychology board contact information

https://doi.org/10.1037/0000448-006
The Neuropsychologist's Workbook: A Hands-On Roadmap to Training and Developing Your Career, by C. Block and S. Hickle

and licensure requirements are also outlined on the American Psychological Association's (APA) organizational website (see https://www.apaservices.org/practice/ce/state/state-info). Especially relevant if you are taking the EPPP while on fellowship: Many state boards meet on a monthly basis to review and approve the materials you submit as part of point b above, the credentials review, but keep in mind that not all do. Look ahead to your specific state's procedures so you factor in the time needed to be reviewed and approved and take the EPPP on your way to licensure.

Once you've decided to take the EPPP, the next important question involves when to take it. In our survey of training directors, two individuals recommended taking it during graduate school, whereas six recommended taking it during internship or in the time between your internship's end and the beginning of your postdoctoral fellowship. A whopping 27 people recommended taking it during your fellowship. At a minimum, you should aim to have both parts completed during the first year (or early in the second year) of your postdoctoral fellowship. Given the range in the responses about when it is best to complete the EPPP, we think it is a valuable question to ask during your graduate, internship, and fellowship interviews. Other frequently asked questions (FAQs) are as follows.

FAQ 1: Where should I begin?

First, take a deep breath and know that more than 80% of test takers pass the EPPP the first time around. This test isn't about trying to learn everything there is to know about psychology because that would simply not be possible. The goal here is to pass, and to achieve that, you must work smarter and not harder. Try to stay away from some third-party websites (i.e., Student-Doctor Network) when preparing to keep yourself at a distance from information that may be incorrect or anxiety-inducing. Familiarize yourself with reliable sources of information, like the chapter on licensure and credentialing in *The Neuropsychologist's Roadmap*. If you want to go more detailed, Association of State & Provincial Psychology Boards has an EPPP candidate handbook that's pretty, well, handy (see https://www.asppb.net/page/CandHandbook).

Then assess what you already know and what you don't. Based on your training, you'll be stronger in some areas than others. We recommend visiting the ASPPB website to scope out pass rates by program, which could inform how well-prepared you may already be. Data are available from years 2015 to 2017 (https://cdn.ymaws.com/www.asppb.net/resource/resmgr/eppp_/2017_Doctoral_Report.pdf), but check back often for any updates. If the scores were high, you can know that your program's curriculum does a good job of preparing you for the exam. You should start with at least one practice exam to judge where you are before any studying takes place, which will also help you determine your knowledge level. For a fee, you can take 200 retired exam questions through the ASPPB website or through a testing center.

We also advise becoming better acquainted with your individual learning style. Now, ascertaining your learning style is not necessarily the most empirical way to go about this, but there is still something valuable to glean from understanding how you best take in information. Check out the learning styles quiz in Table 6.1. Take a moment to check off any statements with which you agree, and sum for each column. Are you an auditory learner? Then you might find studying to be more efficient when listening to recordings of exam questions or study material, listening to relevant podcasts, reading exam questions out loud as well as your answer, coming up with rhymes to learn important information, recording yourself talking through study concepts and models, attending a prep workshop (such as those through study companies such as the Association for Advanced Training in the Behavioral Sciences [AATBS]), or spending time with a study buddy. If you are a visual learner, you might enjoy watching webinars, outlining your notes in a visual format such as tables or graphics, making use of data visualization resources online, or using flashcards or EPPP mobile study apps.

FAQ 2: What should I use to study?

This goes back to what kind of learner you are. Depending on whether you are primarily a visual or auditory learner, this will help you decide what modality to emphasize. That being said, you should consider multimodal studying. By presenting the material across modalities, you're honing your mind to think about the concepts and terms in different ways. This means using a combination of the following: individual review, paired or group review, practice exams, audio files, flashcards, and mobile apps (see Figure 6.1 for example apps at a range of price points).

TABLE 6.1. Learning Styles Quiz

Which statements below do you agree with? Check all that apply.	
☐ I learn best by listening to a lecture.	☐ I learn best by reading a textbook.
☐ I learn by explaining concepts to others.	☐ I learn best by using flashcards.
☐ I remember things I hear more than things I see.	☐ I learn a lot from diagrams and illustrations.
☐ I follow oral directions better than written directions.	☐ I use arrows or other symbols when I take notes.
☐ I sound words out when learning to spell them.	☐ I remember things I see more than things I hear.
☐ I create songs and jingles to remember information.	☐ I prefer teachers who write information on the board.
☐ I read out loud when studying.	☐ I am good at designing graphs, charts, and diagrams.
☐ I learn best when listening to background noise.	☐ When I take a test, I can visualize answers in my head.
☐ I benefit from repeating information to myself.	☐ I like using visual aids like flashcards.
☐ I like listening to podcasts.	☐ I like watching webinars or other visual presentations.
Auditory Learning Total: _____	**Visual Learning Total:** _____

FIGURE 6.1. Examination for Professional Practice in Psychology (EPPP) Mobile Study Apps

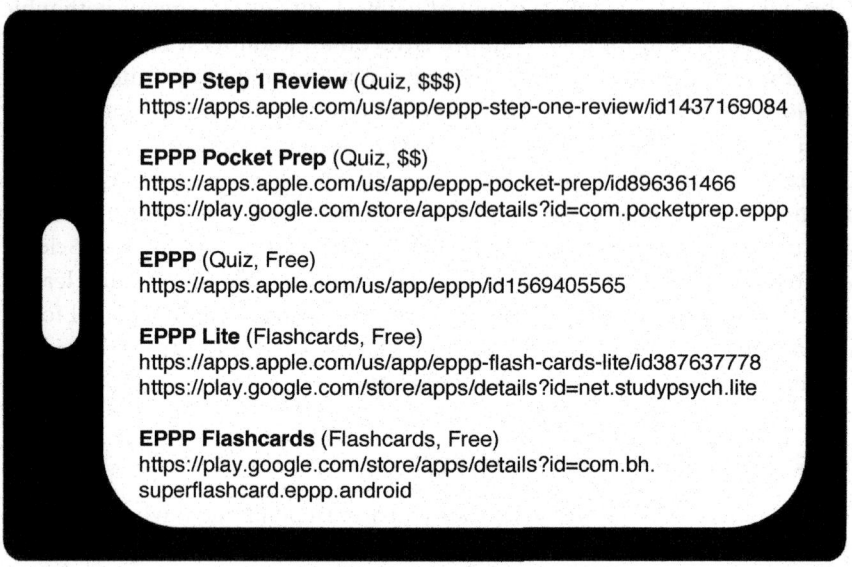

FAQ 3: How "old" can my study materials be?

The beauty of the EPPP (especially Part 1) is that you can use older materials and still do fine because much of the test is based on seminal psychological theories. From the authors' experience, one of us took Part 1 of the EPPP using materials dating back 14 years—and passed with plenty of room to spare. So, bottom line: the materials can be older, and you'll still do fine. In-person workshops and fancy packages are great, but they do cost money. People sell their old materials online all the time (on eBay, for example), which helps offset this. You may also ask around with people you know who have taken or are studying to take the exam and might be willing to part with their old study materials for free or at reduced cost. If taking the EPPP during your fellowship, know that some programs cover the cost of the study materials, so it's worth asking program leadership if this is possible.

FAQ 4: How long should I study?

The amount of time you spend studying does matter for EPPP success—but only up to a certain point. The American Psychological Association has collected some data to this effect (see Clay, 2012). Pass rates are fairly good regardless of which method is employed. You can also see that the pass rate does not appreciably improve after the 200-hour mark, instead declining as the study hours increase. The key is to use your time wisely, and keep in mind that the aim is to pass the test and not to excel on the test (in fact, one could argue that a score well beyond the cutoff reflects study hours that were not necessary).

In our training director survey, respondents' recommended total study time averaged about 80 hours (ranging from as low as 20 to as high as 250). Anecdotally, most people we know who took the first part studied somewhere between 75 and 100 hours. We recommend thinking about how many hours you realistically have available in a given week, let's say 10. Over the course of two and a half months, that adds up to about 100 hours of solid study time.

FAQ 5: How should I study?

This is probably the most important question of all. We authors have heard the gamut of study approaches, ranging from only using practice tests to attending a full-on workshop. We can at least offer our own experience as a point of comparison: We began with a practice test, and then reviewed it to assess strengths and weaknesses. From there, we began to experiment and figure out what did not work versus what did for us.

WHAT DIDN'T WORK?

Dr. Block: I thought I'd start studying by using just the practice tests. The upside to this approach is that the exams more closely approximate the actual testing scenario. The exams are actually designed to be more difficult than the actual exam. People say if you're scoring around 65% correct on your practice exams, then you'll easily pass the real EPPP (Part 1). However, to me this quickly felt like an inefficient way to study. Most practice exams are several hundred questions long, so the review process takes quite a bit of time. I also had more trouble remembering bits of discrete information from all the various questions. It seemed that it would make more sense to start by broadly covering all the essential foundational information, and then following that by filling in knowledge gaps (and applying knowledge) with the practice exams.

Dr. Hickle: I definitely spent too much time studying. I was also told that getting around 65% on the practice exams would be enough to pass the real EPPP, and I was getting those scores on practice exams, but I just didn't feel comfortable with those scores. In the last week before I took the real EPPP, my practice exam scores were probably consistently above 75%, and when I took the exam, I far exceeded the cutoff to pass the actual exam. If I could do it again, I would just trust the data, study less, and be more intentional about my self-care to manage my worries.

WHAT DID WORK?

Dr. Block: I had better luck in switching to reviewing the EPPP PsychPrep book that I had. It had chapters to cover each of the major EPPP test areas. I went through chapter by chapter, one domain at a time. Rather than just passively reading the material, I read and wrote paraphrased notes. I think this helped me to engage more actively with the material. At the same time, I cross-referenced material online when I felt the chapter explained something in less detail than I would have liked or when a concept was still confusing to me. This deepened my knowledge in selected topics and allowed me to better connect material in my head. I supplemented along the way with audio files and mobile apps. Then, the final 1 to 2 weeks before the exam, I did nothing but practice tests and the flashcard apps. This way, I could apply the material I had already learned and fill in the gaps with the exam information. I found the flashcard app to be much more difficult than the quiz app because you had to engage in free recall versus recognition, so by boosting the difficulty level, I was able to master some of the more difficult concepts and terms. As a final note, as psychologists, we all know spaced practice is better than massed practice—apply that rule to yourself during your studies. And be sure to take regular breaks during your study sessions. I found the Pomodoro technique to be quite helpful (including the free online timer on https://pomofocus.io).

Dr. Hickle: My approach to studying worked well for me because it matched my learning style. I took a practice exam first to get a sense of where my strengths and gaps were, as well as the type and specificity of the questions that would be asked. I like to have a good grasp of the foundational material, so I started off listening to the lectures (often in the car during my commute) first. I found the recordings especially helpful for topics that weren't as familiar to me (e.g., I/O). The lectures also had really helpful information, like questions that tend to come up frequently on the exam, mnemonics, and other memory aids. After that, I worked through practice tests, making note of the questions I was getting wrong, reviewing why I was getting it wrong, and then making flashcards.

Once you've decided on an overall approach, the issue then becomes how to tackle the individual test items. Across the EPPP, you will see two types of questions: (a) questions requiring recall of a discrete piece of information and tapping into rote knowledge, such as a question asking about the definition of a specific term, developmental stage, professional standard, or statistical result and (b) questions requiring situational analysis and evaluation, such as an ethical or clinical diagnostic vignette. Here are some suggested test-taking strategies from us:

- Get it out of your head: You are provided with some writing materials in the EPPP exam, typically in the form of a single paper/pencil or dry-erase board. The minute you sit down, take some time to jot down any important information that you want to recall for later.

- Attend to the entire question: The most important thing we can both recommend is to take the time to carefully read the entire item. Note any prefixes or suffixes that may clue you in to the right answer (e.g., a medication with the suffix "zepam" or "zolam" is easily recognized as one in the benzodiazepine class). Be attentive to words and phrases such as "except" or "all but," which are usually prompting for a response that doesn't belong.

And be especially attentive to switchback words like "but," "although," or "nevertheless" which indicate a shift in the nature or focus of the question. You have plenty of time to complete the exam, so it is important that you don't rush yourself and end up missing important details.

- Identify the core element of the question: Exams like the EPPP often throw in extraneous details in questions. After reading the entire question ask yourself, "What exactly are they asking me here?" If the test item is confusing to you, try rephrasing it in your own words.

- Process of elimination: It's impossible to know everything about psychology, so your goal for the EPPP shouldn't be to arrive at one single correct answer for every test item. It's nice when that happens, but it should be the exception and not the expectation. Rather, a good goal for the EPPP is to be able to whittle down every question to the two best answers. In looking at the various answer options, what can you immediately strike from the list? The low-hanging fruit is to look for information that is not relevant to the question at hand. You could also strike from the list any potential similar items. For example:

Which of the following selective serotonin reuptake inhibitors (SSRIs) is often used to treat depression?

A. Sertraline

B. Bupropion

C. Wellbutrin

D. Alprazolam

In this example, we know that we can immediately cross off "D" because alprazolam is a benzodiazepine and not an antidepressant/SSRI. But we can also cross off "B" and "C" because bupropion is not an SSRI and is the generic for Wellbutrin. See how that worked? Some test-taking resources suggest the "+ / − / ?" approach to marking test items, with "+" denoting a possibly correct answer, "−" an incorrect answer, and "?" for any items that you're unsure about.

- Keep it moving: Don't dally too long on any one test item. The exam allows you to skip past questions, flagging them so you can come back to answer later. For anything that isn't immediately answerable, use this approach. It keeps the anxiety to a minimum, and there may even be something later in the exam that triggers recall for one of the items you skipped.

- Confirm your answer: Once you've hit upon your answer, mark it carefully and double-check to make sure. You have plenty of time to do the exam, so no need to rush yourself. You will most likely have plenty of time at the end to review all responses, and we encourage you to do so if possible (but reasonably trust your initial gut response: Second-guessing driven by anticipatory anxiety can sabotage your performance).

- Approach ethics with the standards in mind: Ethics questions warrant a special note here. Ethics questions can be especially tricky because there are shades of gray or other considerations within some of the vignettes presented to you in the exam. We recommend a thorough review of the APA (2017) Ethics Code, and using that to strictly guide your responses rather than basing them on your own clinical training experience. And when in doubt, ask yourself, "What is in the best interest of the patient in this vignette?"

As a final recommendation on studying, we do strongly encourage you to create and use some kind of study tracking tool. Like a true psychologist, collecting data is invaluable for tracking your progress and improvement (see sample log in Table 6.2).

FAQ 6: Should I do anything else?

Yes, don't forget self-care! The EPPP study process can be stress-inducing. You've probably become quite familiar with stress as graduate education/training is, in and of itself, stressful. But add studying on top of a full-time position, and maintaining healthy stress management becomes critical. In a recent study of first-time test-takers, Macura and Ameen (2021) found that 35% of respondents felt that situational demands (including poor self-care and self-defeating beliefs) posed some difficulty in preparing for the EPPP; this was greater than lack of specific coursework in respondents' graduate or internship programs.

We recommend taking a moment to consider your own coping strategies, for better or worse. Are you the kind of person to actively seek social support or find ways to relax your body physically? Conversely, are you the person to be more passively avoidant by binge-watching on your couch? Look at the self-care quiz and plan in Table 6.3. First, think about all the ways you tend to cope with the stress in your life. Check off any that apply, even the less savory ones. Total each of the two columns, and then reflect on what themes emerge. Did you check more positive coping strategies (left column) or negative coping strategies (right column)? Don't skip the written exercise afterward, as it helps to consolidate learning and helps you devise achievable stress management strategies using the SMART goals approach. What does a self-care SMART goal look like? Here is an example: "I will set aside at least 20 to 30 minutes per day, 4 out of 7 days per week, to take a long and hot bubble bath for self-care."

We also encourage you to put to use some of the mindful meditation and relaxation induction techniques you've learned during your training. The 5-4-3-2-1 method or 4-7-8 breathing method are exercises that can help reduce anxiety and stress. *The Neuropsychologist's Roadmap* has a helpful chapter on this topic (Chapter 16). Read it for some additional ideas on self-care and work–life integration.

EPPP PART 2—SKILLS

At the time of this publication, only a handful of states and Canadian provinces have adopted the EPPP2, a licensing exam that is designed to be more of a performance-based (rather than content-based) assessment of skills and

TABLE 6.2. Study Tracking Log

Date	Study or test session?	Topic	Score % correct	Start time	End time	Total hours

Total Study Time

TABLE 6.3. Self-Care Quiz and Plan

How do you cope with stress in general? Check all that apply.	
☐ Spend time with family	☐ Withdraw from others or isolate myself
☐ Spend time with friends	☐ Dive into my work
☐ Clean my desk	☐ Go to sleep
☐ Clean my living space	☐ Overeat or emotionally eat
☐ Stand and stretch	☐ Undereat or starve myself
☐ Make sure I eat healthy	☐ Eat high-fat, high-carb, unhealthy foods
☐ Make sure I eat enough	☐ Drink more than three caffeinated drinks a day
☐ Make sure I sleep 7 to 8 hours at night	
☐ Go for a walk	☐ Drink energy drinks
☐ Go exercise	☐ Use substances like alcohol, tobacco, or drugs
☐ Do a recreational activity or hobby	
☐ Go relax	☐ Overspend or spend impulsively
☐ Rely on my sense of humor	☐ Binge-watch movies or TV shows
☐ Rely on my spirituality	☐ Skip a recreational activity or hobby
☐ Engage in prayer	☐ Be sedentary
☐ Do meditation or deep breathing	☐ Ruminate on my stresses
☐ Do aromatherapy or massage therapy	☐ Feel irritable or snap at others
	☐ Criticize myself
☐ Listen to music	☐ Ignore or avoid what's going on
☐ Watch a feel-good movie or TV show	☐ Catastrophize or jump to conclusions
☐ Attend psychotherapy	☐ Doomscroll
☐ Think positively	☐ Focus on the past
☐ Make plans for the future	☐ Thoughts that life isn't worth living
☐ Reward myself	☐ Self-harm thought or behaviors
	☐ Punish myself

Positive Coping Total: _____   **Negative Coping Total:** _____

What did I learn in this activity? _____

_____

Circle your top three positive coping strategies. Using the SMART goals approach on page 303 of *The Neuropsychologist's Roadmap*, my goals for each of my positive coping strategies include the following:

1) _____

2) _____

3) _____

competencies required for the independent practice of psychology. If you live in and intend to get licensed in one of these regions, here is the information that you should know.

The EPPP2 is designed to evaluate practical skills, such as assessment and diagnosis, treatment planning, intervention implementation, and ethical practice in real-world scenarios. The EPPP2 consists of 170 questions and assesses the following domains: scientific orientation, assessment and intervention, relational competence, professionalism, ethical practice, and collaboration, consultation, and supervision. The EPPP2 is a computer-based exam, just like the EPPP1. Some questions are in the form of a "scenario," where you are given information about a situation (e.g., case example, description of an interview, test protocol). As you answer questions about the scenario, you are presented additional information, and then answer additional questions based on the additional information provided. Other question types are multiple choice (choosing the best choice out of three responses) or multiple choice/ multiple response (i.e., you can choose more than one response from a series of possible answers). You will have 4 hours and 15 minutes to complete the exam. We encourage you to review the ASPPB website for more information about this exam (https://www.asppb.net/page/EPPPPart2-Skills). Appendix C from their EPPP Candidate Handbook provides the competencies that the exam is intended to assess. There is a short video provided by ASPPB providing some sample items on the EPPP2 (ASPPB, 2022). AATBS now offers an exam prep study bundle that includes practice questions, as well as tips and strategies for tackling the exam (https://aatbs.com/psychology/eppp-part-2/online-programs). AATBS also offers an option for you to take a sample exam for $30 per attempt (see https://www.asppb.net/page/eppp2sampleexam).

We spoke to several neuropsychologists and postdoctoral fellows about their experience taking the EPPP2. Everyone characterized the study process as frustrating; at that time, there was so little information about the exam and virtually no resources available to help them study and prepare. A common thread in their advice was to take EPPP2 as quickly as possible after EPPP1 (i.e., within weeks of the first exam) so that the content you studied is still fresh. They also recommended focusing your efforts on studying the domains that overlapped between EPPP1 and 2. They recommended paying particular attention to the APA Ethics Code and crisis management. They also recommended reviewing commonly used measures of personality functioning, as well as measures used in pediatric/child populations, and making sure that you know how to interpret these measures. Five to 15 hours of total study time was considered sufficient to pass. They also noted that the test is especially hard for people who have a tendency to overthink; try not to second-guess yourself and trust your gut.

OTHER STATE EXAMS

Often, states have additional test requirements to be licensed. These may include written and/or oral examinations assessing your knowledge of state-specific rules and laws as well as HIPAA, and in some instances defending a clinical practice sample (e.g., a de-identified neuropsychological report that is submitted to the board). Note that these exams may be virtual, in person, or at a testing center. How do you find a state's particular set of requirements? Easy!

Just search for the psychology board of that state online, or check out this web page: http://psybook.asppb.org. And to which state should you apply, you may then ask? The answer is "it depends." Federal positions, such as those through the Veterans Affairs health care system, require a license, but it doesn't have to be for the state in which you intend to reside or practice. Some other positions don't require licensure at all (e.g., teaching in an academic department at a university). But most other jobs will require a license from the state in which you intend to reside or practice. We encourage you to talk to people who have recently gone through the licensure process and who can provide some guidance. Your supervisors are also good people to ask for advice and support.

CONTINUING EDUCATION

Now that you have your license, you have to work to maintain it over time. This is done through completion of continuing education, informally called CEs. CEs are expressed in credit units ranging from 0.5 and up, with higher values reflecting more time invested in a given learning experience (e.g., a 90-minute lecture is typically worth 1.5 CE credits). The number of CE credits required to maintain your license varies by state, with some requiring more than others or documentation more often than others. In Georgia, for instance, licenses are renewed every 2 years, and 40 CEs must be earned during that period of time. Alabama, on the other hand, requires 20 CEs per year. We recommend Googling "psychology board CE requirements" for a few different states to get a sense of how state requirements vary. Some states now require that a certain portion of CEs earned each year must relate to ethics or cultural competency/diversity.

How do you obtain CEs? There are many ways to do this. Common ones include attending lectures at conferences, attending online webinars, attending educational events at your institution (e.g., grand rounds), reading books, reading journal articles, or by reading some professional magazine articles (e.g., APA's *Monitor on Psychology*). Some states allow you to count publishing journal articles or books/book chapters, teaching courses, or becoming board certified toward your CE requirements. As of 2023, earning your American Board of Professional Psychology certification in clinical neuropsychology counted for 40 CE credits! It's important to note that CEs must come from an approved continuing education provider such as the APA or Accreditation Council for Continuing Medical Education. Keep tidy records: You will need to maintain copies of the CE completion certificates you receive and track your credits to ensure you've completed a sufficient quantity (while satisfying special ethics or diversity requirements). State boards do conduct routine member audits, so you want to ready in case that happens! For tracking purposes, we recommend using a tracking log similar to Table 6.4. We recommend that you create a folder (a paper copy or an electronic one on your computer) and save all your completion certificates and your tracking log there so they are easily accessed if you do get audited.

TABLE 6.4. Continuing Education (CE) Tracking Log (Sample)

Year	Category	Event	Title	CEs
2023	General	Neurology grand rounds	Long COVID: Cognition	3.00
2023	Ethics	APA Convention	Ethics of Supervision	1.50
2023	General	INS online webinar	Antiseizure Medications	2.00
2023	Diversity	APA *Monitor* article	Cultural Interviews	0.50
2023	General	ABPP	Board Certification	40.00
Total				47.00

Note. ABPP = American Board of Professional Psychology; APA = American Psychological Association; CEs = continuing education credits; INS = International Neuropsychological Society.

CREDENTIALING

There are a couple types of credentialing. One type is the credentialing conferred by professional bodies. This simply means that you meet specific educational and training eligibility criteria set out by a given professional body. Certainly, there are an array of professional credentials granted by other groups such as the Certified Brain Injury Specialist credential through the Brain Injury Association of America (https://www.biausa.org). Two examples of this in professional psychology are credentials through the National Register for Health Service Psychologists (https://www.nationalregister.org) and the National Association of School Psychology (https://www.nasponline.org).

Then, there is the credentialing that you do once you're hired as a neuropsychologist in a health care setting. This credentialing means that your training/educational background and license have been verified and you have been granted privileges to (a) practice in your institution and (b) become "paneled" with various health insurance companies—meaning that you are a recognized and accepted provider by each company, which allows you to bill and be reimbursed for any services that you provide. The ability to practice comes after completion of licensure, which is governed and regulated by the ASPPB (https://www.asppb.net). Paneling, on the other hand, is slightly different. In some settings, it can be lengthy or complex, like if you are in a private practice setting, which can require you to manage this process yourself (although you could instead hire a third-party business to do this for you). In other settings, the credentialing process can be easy or even nonexistent; for example, VA hospitals don't bill for insurance, so no paneling is necessary. If in an institutional setting such as an academic medical center or private hospital, it's a little easier because hospitals have departments and staff that manage this for providers. You will be asked to do a couple of things:

1. Apply for a provider identification number called the National Provider Identifier Standard, or NPI for short. This is a unique 10-digit number that all covered health care providers must obtain, including neuropsychologists. These are used in standard transactions such as health insurance claims for services that you render to patients. You apply for the NPI through a federally

managed system called the National Plan and Provider Enumeration System (https://npiregistry.cms.hhs.gov). Applying is free, and the online form usually takes a half hour or less. And if you happen to lose your NPI, you can easily look it up online.

2. Once you have your NPI, you will need to submit any requested materials to your institution's privileging or credentialing office. This includes submitting personal identifying information such as your name and date of birth, NPI number, a copy of your state psychology license, board certification (if you have it), practice/employer information, CV, transcripts, personal and academic references, and proof of liability/malpractice insurance (although hospitals generally manage this part). Your institution will take this information and submit applications on your behalf to the US Centers for Medicare and Medicaid Services (CMS) as well as private payors such as Blue Cross/ Blue Shield, Aetna, Cigna, and others.

Once you have submitted your application to CMS or a private payor, it goes through a few additional steps: (a) CMS or the private payor will process the application, (b) verify your credentials, and (c) send it to their credentialing committee for approval. It is very important to verify that all information you submit during the credentialing process is correct because one tiny error could set you back for months. Although the application portion of the credentialing process can be fairly quick, ranging anywhere from 30 to 90 days, once approved, the provider must go through a contracting phase, and that can add another 30 days (making total possible time from application to finalized contract being anywhere from 90 to 120 days).

You might now see why we so strongly emphasize early completion of the EPPP process. If you wait too long, it delays completion of your state license which then delays completion of the credentialing process, potentially pushing back your job's start date, but almost certainly drawing the ire of your immediate supervisor. A good rule of thumb here is to just get it done or, as Dr. Block puts it, "eat that frog." If you're confused about why she recommends dining on an amphibian, her advice stems from productivity consultant Brian Tracy's (2017) *Eat That Frog*, which was inspired by this quote by Mark Twain: "If it's your job to eat a frog, it's best to do it first thing in the morning. And if it's your job to eat two frogs, it's best to eat the biggest one first."

In short, seek to complete your biggest, most important task first. If you have more than one of them sitting on your to do list, start with the biggest/ hardest/most important one first. Not many people enjoy sinking time into the minutiae of application paperwork, but credentialing is an important prerequisite to practicing neuropsychology (and getting paid) so "eat that frog" and get the EPPP done early. Once you have your license and you're credentialed, you can relax, right? Well, not quite. There is one more step in your journey to becoming a neuropsychologist: board certification. We'll cover that in the next chapter.

7

Board Certification in Neuropsychology

 Before working through activities on this topic, be sure to read through Chapter 5 of *The Neuropsychologist's Roadmap*.

This chapter is all about getting board certification. This is the step that demonstrates your expertise and competence in the field of neuropsychology. There are several certifications in neuropsychology in the United States, and they typically involve a combination of education, supervised clinical experience, and successful completion of examinations. Chapter 5 of *The Neuropsychologist's Roadmap* (Block, 2021) delves into what board certification is and the benefits of being board certified in further detail than we'll do here, but this workbook can serve as a helpful study and organizational companion during the process. We will also provide some helpful advice and recommendations from 28 board-certified neuropsychologists who gave us their thoughts on how best to prepare for each of these steps, the resources they used, and how to avoid potential holdups in the board-certification process.

WHERE AND WHEN TO BEGIN

Begin by considering whether board certification is right for you. We are strong proponents for board certification, and our personal bias is that neuropsychology trainees should plan for this. But we do acknowledge that there are some jobs (i.e., teaching and doing research in an academic department) in which board certification is less beneficial, and so time may be better spent accruing publications or other relevant experiences.

https://doi.org/10.1037/0000448-007

The Neuropsychologist's Workbook: A Hands-On Roadmap to Training and Developing Your Career, by C. Block and S. Hickle

Next, familiarize yourself with existing resources. Again, we recommend the chapter on board certification (Chapter 5) in *The Neuropsychologist's Roadmap*. Exhibit 5.1 on page 94 of that chapter provides an overview of each of the steps, fees, and materials needed, and Table 5.2 on page 101 provides general guidance and resources to help you prepare for each of these steps. The *Board Certification in Clinical Neuropsychology* book by Armstrong et al. (2019) is also an excellent resource that provides an overview of the process of becoming board certified.

When should you start preparing? When we asked survey respondents for their top piece of advice for people embarking on the board-certification process, the overwhelming response was "just do it." Many commented how the longer you wait, the harder it becomes. And if you're waiting for the perfect time, don't! One neuropsychologist commented, "There is no perfect time. You will only get busier in your job (and family life) over time, so just get it done as early as possible." Multiple people recommended starting right after completing your postdoctoral fellowship (if possible) since you are still in the "training mode" mindset (and perhaps even fresh out of a neuroanatomy course as part of your fellowship). If you are worried that this is too early in your career and that you haven't amassed enough clinical experience to pass, don't be. Even seasoned clinicians with a wealth of experience still need to study. You're actually at a bit of an advantage: A recent study showed that persons still within the 10-year period after completing their doctorate degree (what we call "early career") passed the oral portion of the board exam process at a significantly higher rate than those past the early career phase (86% vs. 69%; Bordes Edgar et al., 2019). So try to start as soon as possible, set a goal date for you to be board certified, and then work backward from that.

When should you set your target date? Although you are allowed 7 years to complete the entire board-certification process, the neuropsychologists that we surveyed told us that it took them about 3 years on average. Exactly 50% of the people we surveyed took less than 3 years, and the minimum amount of time taken for the full process was 1 year. Whenever you do begin, we recommend that you give yourself 1 to 2 years to finish the entire process— and do everything in your power to stick to that deadline.

THE APPLICATION AND CREDENTIAL REVIEW

Recall from Chapter 5 of *The Neuropsychologist's Roadmap* that the entire board-certification examination process includes three components: a written portion, practice sample submission, and oral portion (see Figure 7.1). The application and credential review process precedes all of these. Using our American Board of Professional Psychology (ABPP) example to get a better sense of the application and credentialing process, you can visit their website, which details all of this nicely (https://abpp.org/application-information/application-process). In short, there are two steps. Step one involves a general credential review by the central office at ABPP and covers your training background, internship training, and licensure status (this is why it's important to keep good records

FIGURE 7.1. The Board Certification Journey

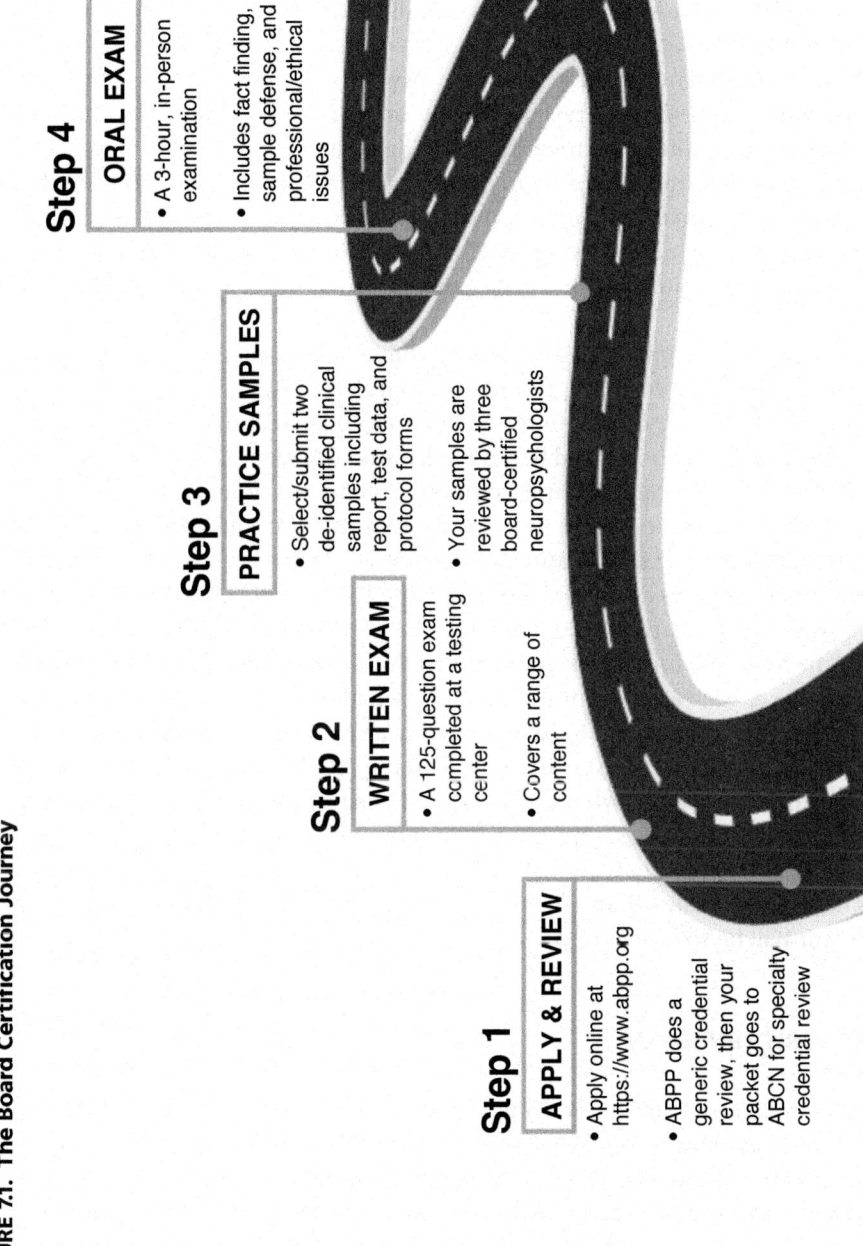

Step 1

APPLY & REVIEW

- Apply online at https://www.abpp.org

- ABPP does a generic credential review, then your packet goes to ABCN for specialty credential review

Step 2

WRITTEN EXAM

- A 125-question exam completed at a testing center

- Covers a range of content

Step 3

PRACTICE SAMPLES

- Select/submit two de-identified clinical samples including report, test data, and protocol forms

- Your samples are reviewed by three board-certified neuropsychologists

Step 4

ORAL EXAM

- A 3-hour, in-person examination

- Includes fact finding, sample defense, and professional/ethical issues

Note. ABCN = American Board of Clinical Neuropsychology; ABPP = American Board of Professional Psychology.

and use the ABPP early-entry option we mention in Chapter 5 of this workbook). Once the first step is passed, your application is forwarded on to the American Board of Clinical Neuropsychology (ABCN) for a specialty credentials review. To confirm the successful completion of specialty-specific training requirements. Note that ABCN requires training conforming to the Houston Conference guidelines (https://uh.edu/hns/hc.html), including a 2-year postdoctoral fellowship with (briefly summarized, see the ABCN website for more detail): (a) at least 50% of time devoted to neuropsychology training; (b) didactics across eight core knowledge areas including basic neurosciences, functional neuroanatomy, neuropathology, clinical neurology, psychological assessment, clinical neuropsychological assessment, psychopathology, and psychological intervention; and (c) supervision by one or more on-site clinical neuropsychologists. Applicants not meeting eligibility criteria may need to complete formal respecialization training in neuropsychology. Anyone concerned that they might not meet eligibility criteria is encouraged to contact the board, with contact information being listed on the frequently asked questions page on the ABCN website (https://theabcn.org/credential-review-frequently-asked-questions).

As you are wrapping up this step, we have several pieces of advice. First, begin planning out your rough timeline/goal to complete each step. Having a reasonable and clear completion timeline in mind can allow you to maintain focus in your progress toward board certification. As you plan ahead, you can consider your clinical load and competing demands as you schedule your exam dates. Are there certain times of the year that are a little lighter in terms of your clinical load? Do fall and winter seasons tend to be crazy due to family and school activities and holidays? Knowing that it will be harder to keep to a study schedule during these busy times can help you be judicious in planning the best time for you to study and set your exam. Second piece of advice: Have others hold you accountable. Tell your family members, colleagues, mentors, and anyone else to help you stick to your plan. Third, start looking for practice sample cases starting Day 1 on the job. We have a section later in this chapter devoted to what makes a good versus bad sample case. This way, you have your practice samples ready to submit right after passing the written exam, and you can keep the ball rolling without losing any steam. We know it's hard to find time when you are in a demanding setting, but accomplishing this feat will be so worth it!

THE WRITTEN EXAM

You've received your letter congratulating you on passing the credential review, which means you are eligible to register for the written exam. Take a deep breath and approach the next step with confidence, especially if you've had solid training in neuropsychology, great didactics, and a good breadth of clinical cases. To be clear, you do have to study, but you've got an excellent foundation already. Many people have told us that studying for the written exam, while arduous, was helpful and even at times enjoyable because it's so much more relevant for clinical practice than the Examination for Professional Practice in Psychology (EPPP).

As far as when to take the exam, we recommend scheduling your exam for 3 to 6 months out. If you schedule your exam farther out than that, you're going to get burnt out from studying, and you'll just end up forgetting information. Our survey respondents indicated that they spent an average of 130 hours studying (standard deviation of 97), with quite a large range (40 to 400 hours total, although we note that 400 hours was a statistical outlier). Fifty percent of our survey respondents studied 100 hours or less, and 75% of our survey respondents studied 162 hours or less, so we think 130 hours is a more than reasonable estimate for how much time to devote to your studies. If you squeeze 130 hours into 3 months of studying, that amounts to around 11 hours per week. If you decide to stretch studying into 6 months, that amounts to about 5 or 6 hours per week. Figure out which is feasible for you. And remember, you don't have to study everything in one chunk of time during the week. Actually, we recommend that you space out your studies so you can learn and retain the information longer. So could you study every Saturday for 4 hours, and then spend an hour every other day of the week reviewing your flashcards?

As far as what resources to use for your studies, the *Clinical Neuropsychology Study Guide and Board Review* by Stucky et al. (2020) is frequently mentioned as a great aid to prepare for the written exam. We had neuropsychologists call it "the single best resource," and recommended that people "live, eat, sleep and breathe" this text. On the basis of our own conversations with people who took the written exam in recent years, this is the one we would choose as a core text. Many successful candidates then deepen their knowledge of specific content areas with chapters from other textbooks (for a list of recommended books and other study materials, see Figure 7.2). We do want to emphasize that it is not the best use of your time to read all of these other textbooks cover to cover. For instance, Blumenfeld's (2021) *Neuroanatomy Through Clinical Cases* will go into much more depth than is necessary for the exam. But if you find that you are struggling with stroke syndromes and keep getting those questions wrong on practice exams, you can read through the chapter on the cerebral hemispheres and vascular supply in more detail.

We would recommend creating a study schedule to ensure you can get through all the material (e.g., chapters from Stucky et al., 2020), and intersperse your studying with practice exams so you can get a pulse on the domains that are weaknesses for you. There are a couple of sample schedules and mock exams on the *Be Ready for ABPP in Neuropsychology* (BRAIN; https://brainaacn. org/) website. Use the strategies that have worked for you in the past—for instance, what worked when you were studying for the EPPP. Try to use active study methods as much as possible rather than passive reading; active study methods include things like taking notes; highlighting text; creating tables, figures, or flowcharts to summarize information; creating flashcards; creating your own multiple-choice questions; and linking the material that

FIGURE 7.2. Resources for the Written Exam

**Be Ready for ABPP in Neuropsychology website -
https://brainaacn.org/**
The Little Black Book of Neuropsychology (Schoenberg & Scott, 2011)
Neuropsychological Assessment (5th ed.; Lezak et al., 2012)
Neuroanatomy Through Clinical Cases (3rd ed.; Blumenfeld, 2021)
Textbook of Clinical Neuropsychology (2nd ed.; Morgan & Ricker, 2018)
Clinical Neuropsychology: A Pocket Handbook for Assessment (4th ed.; Parsons & Braun, 2024)
Pediatric Neuropsychology: Research, Theory, and Practice (3rd ed.; Beauchamp et al., 2022)
Clinical Neuropsychology (5th ed.; Heilman & Valenstein, 2012)
Conducting a Culturally Informed Neuropsychological Evaluation (Fujii, 2016)
Developmental Neuropsychology: A Clinical Approach (2nd ed.; Anderson et al., 2019)
Ethical Principles of Psychologists and Code of Conduct (APA, 2017)

Note. ABPP = American Board of Professional Psychology.

you are learning to cases that you are seeing. Remember to take practice exams under timed circumstances so you can better approximate the actual examination!

Many people tout the benefits of joining a group to study. You can request to join a study group on the BRAIN website, where you will be grouped with other individuals preparing for the written exam at the same time. Don't feel coerced to join if you're not a group study person. However, you should note the benefits before passing up an opportunity to join a study group. First, you'll have more people holding you accountable to study. It is so easy to tell yourself that you'll skip this week and just get back into it the next week when you've got a busy clinical week if you are studying alone. The (hopefully friendly) peer pressure can help you stay on track. Also, different members of the group may have different training backgrounds and areas of expertise that can help fill gaps in your understanding and expose you to materials you might have missed.

We know that this seems like a lot of material to study. Per the ABCN manual, there are specific content areas that are covered by the exam. These include (a) general psychology (including statistics and methodology), (b) general clinical psychology, (c) general psychopathology/neuropathology, (d) brain–behavior relationships, and (e) the practice of clinical neuropsychology. Questions may cover factual, historical, practice, and/or professional issues, including ethics and individual/cultural diversity. To get a better understanding of the scope and the depth of the questions that you may be asked, we recommend taking a practice exam at the beginning (before you start studying). It's also a great way to assess the domains and areas that are weak for you. You are not expected to and can't possibly know everything, so think big picture. Try not to get too into the weeds of the details on any topic—you're not going to be asked about zebras or incredibly obscure information. If you find that you are getting too granular in your studies, ask yourself how you might be able to apply these concepts within the context of everyday clinical work. If you are unable to see a clear link, you have probably gone too far. Relatedly, don't overstudy topics that you already know well. Be prepared to answer questions about differential diagnosis and functional neuroanatomy. Also, don't forget to study other topics that may not seem as apparent—like ethics, psychometrics, rehabilitation, research-supported recommendations/interventions, and cultural considerations. For our pediatric neuropsychologists studying for the written exam, our advice for you is to really study up on different dementia etiologies, delirium, and medication classes for older adults.

When taking the exam, similar to the EPPP make sure you're familiar with the testing center location and give yourself plenty of time to arrive (bringing any required documents with you). Try to calm your nerves. Realistically, you will not know all the answers. No matter how much you studied, there will be times when you will have to shrug and move on because you never covered that topic in your studies. This is normal. Don't let it throw you. There's really no way to know everything about psychology and neuropsychology; the idea is to have sufficient knowledge to be able to approach the test with a reasonable strategy.

Chapter 6's FAQ 5 provides test-taking strategies that you can also use when taking the written exam. Just like the EPPP, the written exam is a multiple-choice test. Read the questions carefully, eliminate obviously wrong answers, and manage your time carefully. Of note, you will have some scratch paper/a small whiteboard during the exam. Before you look at any questions, "brain dump" all those facts that you are worried you'll forget—cranial nerves, statistics formulas, mnemonics for genetic conditions, drawings of the visual pathway, and so on. You may even consider practicing what you will write down in the week leading up to the exam so you can do this that much more quickly on the day of.

THE PRACTICE SAMPLE

Once you receive the news that you have passed your written exam (typically several weeks after you've taken it), you will be invited to submit two work samples. We've provided a list of do's and don'ts to consider as you make your case selection (see Table 7.1). Generally, you want to remember that you are demonstrating competence, not your cutting-edge expertise. You don't want to pick a case that is a spectacularly low base-rate condition, just because it's interesting. Pick cases that you see often within the scope of your normal practice and demonstrate your skill, where you really feel like you nailed it.

On the other end, know that there will never be a perfect case. Consider sending your samples to senior colleagues who are familiar with the board-certification process, and they can give you feedback as to whether they believe

TABLE 7.1. Case Selection Do's and Don'ts

Do	Don't
✓ Have a clear neurological underpinning and demonstrate your knowledge of brain–behavior relationships (i.e., the data correlate with the neuropathology/area of brain injury)	✗ Pick an overly complex case—cases that have multiple etiologies, confounding factors, or require a lot of rule-outs and differentials
✓ Have a complete/comprehensive (not necessarily exhaustive) battery	✗ Pick a "cool" or "zebra" case just because it is interesting
✓ Have a good history and incorporate some collateral information	✗ Pick cases with controversial topics (e.g., chronic traumatic encephalopathy, nonverbal learning disability, COVID-19)
✓ Pick cases that are fairly clear-cut and relatively straightforward (i.e., data and histories align in a clear way)	✗ Pick cases that raise ethical concerns about your practice
✓ Pick "bread-and-butter" cases that showcase the types of patients you commonly see in practice	✗ Pick cases where there is no pattern of low scores to interpret (i.e., no cognitive impairment)
✓ Have diagnoses that a majority of neuropsychologists would readily agree on	✗ Pick cases where there the impairment is so severe and global that it does not show off your interpretation skills
✓ Pick cases that are a good representation of your knowledge and skills	✗ Pick cases where you lack expertise
✓ Explore differential diagnoses, where readers can walk through your line of reasoning for the conceptualization	✗ Pick cases where anything in the clinical picture doesn't make sense to you
✓ Demonstrate clear and concise writing, and includes evidence-based and patient-specific recommendations	✗ Pick cases where psychological, mood, or personality disorders are the primary factors
	✗ Pick cases with controversial diagnoses or recommendations

your work samples are good ones to submit. If you don't have any mentors or colleagues whom you could ask to do this for you, you can submit a request for a mentor through the mentorship match program sponsored by AACN/BRAIN (https://theabcn.org/mentorship-program).

Also, know that you will have the opportunity to provide some more context and reasoning to your case samples in a "Supporting Information" document. You are allowed three pages maximum. For instance, if there were test results that were unusual/atypical, or you wanted the reviewers to know the differentials that you considered and ruled out (but did not include this within your report for whatever reason), this is the place to explain your reasoning. As a last step, review the checklist (Exhibit 7.1) to ensure you have completed everything prior to submission.

THE ORAL EXAM

There's just one last hurdle: the oral exam. Although this one does seem to cause some anxiety in test takers, feel reassured that the pass rates for the oral exam are actually higher than the written exam and may require less preparatory

EXHIBIT 7.1

Sample Submission Checklist

Tasks

Case 1

☐ Review the data summary sheet and raw test protocols to ensure that all tests were scored correctly and appropriate norms were applied.

☐ Remove your name and institutional information (including institution name, location, and any provider information) from your final report, data summary sheet, and raw test protocols—don't forget to check headers and footers!

☐ Remove patient information from your final report, data summary sheet, and raw test protocols—don't forget to check headers and footers!

☐ Save as one PDF file.

Case 2

☐ Review the data summary sheet and raw test protocols to ensure that all tests were scored correctly and appropriate norms were applied.

☐ Remove your name and institutional information (including institution name, location, and any provider information) from your final report, data summary sheet, and raw test protocols—don't forget to check headers and footers!

☐ Remove patient information from your final report, data summary sheet, and raw test protocols—don't forget to check headers and footers!

☐ Save as one PDF file.

General

☐ Have a trusted person double-check that your two practice samples are indeed de-identified.

☐ Consider taking advantage of the optional supporting information document, which can be up to three pages and include contextual information to help your reviewers and oral examiner better understand your practice samples (e.g., norms used, diagnostic considerations, limitations, supporting references).

☐ Prepare your professional data sheet, which it typically one or two pages and should include your name, professional position, education, clinical populations served, and an activity breakdown of how your time is currently spent.

☐ Submit your practice samples online.

time. In our survey, people on average studied for 46 hours (plus or minus 41 hours). Half of our sample studied 30 hours or fewer, while 75% of our sample studied 50 hours or fewer. You'll still have to prepare, however, so we've got some advice for you on how you can spend this time wisely. We've also included a list of resources that were cited as helpful by board-certified neuropsychologists (Figure 7.3).

The oral exam itself is proprietary, and for antispoilage purposes we cannot go into much detail about what the specific day will look like. We can, however,

FIGURE 7.3. Resources for the Oral Exam

Be Ready for ABPP in Neuropsychology website - https://brainaacn.org
The Neuropsychology Fact-Finding Casebook: A Training Resource (Stucky & Bush, 2017)
Ethical Decision Making in Clinical Neuropsychology (2nd ed.; Bush, 2007)
A Casebook of Ethical Challenges in Neuropsychology (Bush, 2005)
Casebook of Clinical Neuropsychology (Morgan et al., 2011)
Conducting a Culturally Informed Neuropsychological Evaluation (Fujii, 2016)
Ethical Principles of Psychologists and Code of Conduct (APA, 2017)
National Academy of Neuropsychology Position Papers
American Academy of Clinical Neuropsychology Official Position Papers and Statements

Note. ABPP = American Board of Professional Psychology.

provide some study and preparation tips, which we've done below, broken down by oral exam component. But before delving into the exam, we do want to acknowledge that part of exam preparation is adequately managing test anxiety. We want to normalize that feeling anxious is normal and something experienced by many examinees. You don't want test anxiety to be the determining factor in whether you pass or fail. Remind yourself: You've come this far, and this step of the process is really just showing the examiners what you already do every single day. Remind yourself of the high pass rate. Make sure you seek emotional and social support along the way and know that it's okay to seek help if you find the anxiety becoming difficult to manage.

As a final note, the oral exam is an in-person exam that requires travel to either Dallas, TX (spring) or Chicago, IL (fall). Plan your trip with ample time: Avoid flying late the night before to mitigate potential airline delays, lost luggage, and the stress of last-minute arrangements. Get there a day or two early to allow you to adjust to the time zone. Don't cram the night before; it is vastly more important to try to get a good night's sleep before the exam (and eat a nutritious breakfast on the day of). Alternatively, there is a form that you can fill out if you would like to request a virtual examination—but this must be approved by the board, and there are a very limited set of circumstances and reasons for when this would be allowed.

The Fact-Finding Portion

First, we recommend creating a solid outline/template that you can use to structure your approach when you are asking questions and soliciting test data from each domain. This is something you can fit onto a single piece of paper that will allow you to go on autopilot on the day of the exam. It's easy to forget about medications, developmental history, previous neuropsychological revaluations, lab work, and other factors when the pressure is on. We have provided what is probably an overly thorough fact-finding outline in Exhibit 7.2, and you can use this to help guide your practice. There is also a sample fact-finding outline on the BRAIN website.

EXHIBIT 7.2

Fact Finding Outline

Referral Reason, History/Background, and Clinical Interview

Demographics
    Age
    Sex
    Race/ethnicity
    Handedness
    Years of education
    Language (primary language, monolingual vs. multilingual)

Referral information
    Referring provider specialty
    Reason for referral
    Patient's own goals for evaluation

Current level of functioning (from patient and collateral report)
    Cognitive: type, onset, course, patient insight into cognitive issues
    Functional status: for basic activities versus instrumental activities, compensatory
        strategies/aids used
    Physical: sensory, gross and fine motor, appetite/dietary preferences, weight, pain,
        sleep, fatigue
    Emotional: mood, personality/behavior changes, hallucinations, delusions, suicidality,
        treatment

Medical records review
    Labs/bloodwork
    Neuroimaging findings
    Prior cognitive screening or neuropsychological evaluation
    Medications and supplements

History/background
    Patient medical and psychiatric history
    Family medical and psychiatric history
    Birth/developmental history
    Educational history
    Occupational history
    Psychosocial history
    Substance use/abuse history
    Legal history

(continues)

EXHIBIT 7.2

Fact Finding Outline (*Continued*)

Evaluation observations
   Arrival/appearance
   Sensory function (limitations, use of aids)
   Motor function (limitations, use of aids)
   Alertness/orientation
   Mood/affect
   Speech/language
   Thought process/content
   Approach to examiner and testing
   Task engagement

Test Results

Sensory and motor function
Premorbid estimation
Global cognition
Intellectual functioning
Academic achievement
Speech and language
Visuospatial and constructional skills
Processing speed
Attention and working memory
Verbal learning/memory
Nonverbal/visual learning/memory
Executive functioning
Self-report inventories (mood, personality, behavior, pain, sleep, quality of life)
Collateral inventories (mood, personality, behavior, adaptive function)

Once you have a solid template in place: practice, practice, practice. Then practice some more. Complete as many fact findings as you can. We find *The Neuropsychology Fact-Finding Casebook* by Stucky and Bush (2017) to be an excellent resource for studying (and if you're reading this well ahead of board certification, we advise you to hold off purchasing this book until you reach that step so as not to spoil this precious resource). Practice with a combination of folks—supervisors, peers, or someone you don't know very well. This diversity prepares you for various dynamics you might face during the actual exam. Consider having boarded supervisors be tough (and even) unfair on you when you practice. It toughens you up for the real deal. And try to practice without your outline—you won't have access to any materials because you can't bring it with you for this portion of the exam. So use the first couple of minutes to organize your thoughts and write down your outline on a blank piece of paper. As you do more fact-finding, you may find that you have to adjust your outline. This is good! It means you are fine-tuning your outline so your approach is even more effective when you take the actual exam. The more you practice, the more confident you will become.

Time management is one hurdle for many people. Fact-finding moves faster than you think! Limit yourself to 45 to 50 minutes during practice sessions to simulate the time pressure of the actual exam (leaving at least 10 of those minutes for your final summary, diagnosis, and recommendations plus any questions the examiner may have). This ensures you can efficiently complete the entire fact-finding process within the allotted timeframe. As you go, jot down quick notes on all the possible etiologies that fit the emerging clinical picture. An acronym such as VINDICATE (Table 7.2) can often be useful to learn, as it helps you work through the most pertinent potential etiologies. By the time you reach your summary step, you should be able to summarize what you've gleaned so far. We suggest touching on the following:

1. Any discrepancy between premorbid and current cognitive functioning.

2. Lateralization versus localization or focal versus multifocal patterns of impairment and what brain regions are involved, using psychometric and behavioral and historical data to support.

3. The neuropsychological profile in terms of pattern analysis (cortical vs. subcortical, strengths vs. weaknesses, prominent vs. lesser deficits—however you want to slice and dice it).

4. Overall severity of impairment and associated neurocognitive diagnosis.

5. Underlying etiology that the history and results are most consistent with (noting both primary and secondary contributors), including a few rule-outs of things that are close considerations or clear rule-outs.

6. Functional implications (e.g., work, driving, school, decision-making).

7. Relevant recommendations.

As you practice, find a pause point and listen to one of the mock fact-finding sessions produced by the Navigating Neuropsychology podcast series. There are three episodes thus far, and likely more to come over time: #109 (https://www.navneuro.com/109), #113 (https://www.navneuro.com/113), and #125

TABLE 7.2. VINDICATE Acronym

Vascular	AVM, stroke, CVD, amyloid angiopathy
Infection	Meningitis, viral encephalitis
Neoplasm	Primary brain tumor, paraneoplastic
Degenerative	AD, VD, DLB, PD, PD+, FTD, HD, Prion disease, HIV
Iatrogenic/Idiopathic	Psychiatric, functional neurological, epilepsy
Congenital	Genetic or developmental conditions
Autoimmune	MS, SLE, CNS autoimmune
Trauma	TBI
Endocrine/Environment	Substance abuse, toxic exposure

Note. AD = Alzheimer's disease; AVM = arteriovenous malformation; CNS = central nervous system; CVD = cardiovascular disease; DLB = dementia with Lewy bodies; FTD = frontotemporal dementia; HD = Huntington Disease; MS = multiple sclerosis; PD = Parkinson's disease; PD+ = Parkinson-plus syndrome; SLE = systemic lupus erythematosus; TBI = traumatic brain injury; VD = vascular disease.

(https://www.navneuro.com/125). You may find these quite helpful in guiding your own approach and practice.

On the day of the exam, all that time spent creating and memorizing your outline should benefit you. Spend the first 5 minutes writing down all this information. As you solicit questions regarding the background history and review/integrate scores, think out loud as you go. More than you think you should. Your examiner should be able to follow (and hence hear) your thought process. We also advise that you have a section reserved on your piece of paper for information that you need to ask about later, and a section for jotting down recommendations as you think of them during the exam. Do not wait until the end to integrate your data and provide your conceptualization. It may help to pretend that you are teaching someone, so that you keep verbalizing what you are thinking. Explain your reasoning for why you are asking the questions that you are and how you are thinking through the conceptualization. Try to answer in a way that demonstrates your knowledge of brain–behavior relationships.

You will have to solicit each domain of cognition, behavior, and emotion, and each of these will be provided on a separate piece of paper. Remember that your examiner will only hand you what you ask for. Also, if you do not know a certain test measure, you can ask! You are not expected to know every measure, and examiners will give you more information about the measure. Further, you may not necessarily be presented with percentiles and certainly not with qualitative descriptors; therefore, make you study these and commit them memory.

During the fact-finding, be sure to pay attention to the time! In an attempt to be thorough, there is a tendency to linger on the history section in particular; however, this can backfire and leave you scrambling when the time comes to summarize, diagnose, and provide recommendations. We recommend that you keep your questions broad (e.g., "Please provide the educational history" rather than "What kinds of grades did they get in school?"). And try not to keep asking the same question multiple times if you have already been given an answer. If your examiner says, "You now have all of the information related to XYZ," trust them and move on. It is also worth noting that your examiner may sometimes interrupt you. Know that this is not meant to be rude; rather, this is an attempt to keep things running on time so you have sufficient time to let all your wonderful knowledge and skills shine!

The Practice Sample Defense

It is important to know your cases inside and out. And be mindful that anything and everything in your report is fair game for questioning. You included EEG results in your report? They're left-handed? Bilingual? Have a family history of depression? They have other medical conditions that you included in the medical history section? Yep, you can be asked about that. Immerse yourself in the empirical literature associated with your diagnoses—think recent literature reviews and meta-analyses. Don't forget to study the neuroanatomy, neurotransmitters, and neuropathology of your diagnoses, etiologies, syndromes, as well as similar diagnoses. Know the indications of medications, and whether they increase risk for cognitive side effects. Be able to defend the choice of all the assessments and the norms that you used.

Anticipate questions and prepare answers to those questions. The best way to address the questions that can be asked about is to send your samples to colleagues and ask them to review the reports with a magnifying glass and note questions that you could be asked or areas to prepare to discuss. Try to find someone with agonizingly high standards (preferably someone outside your direct supervisory line) and ask them to read your samples and generate questions. Seek out people in your network who have expertise in that specific population and ask them to provide their criticisms as well as questions they would ask if they were the examiner. They may help you think through reasonable responses to tricky questions or provide specific resources for you to review as you prepare. Your goal is to be able to anticipate as many questions as reasonably possible based on the samples provided and practice answering those questions until it becomes second nature. Don't forget to think about questions that you may be asked about potential ethical scenarios on your case samples—think issues related to third-party observers and test security issues. Remember to review the position papers (see Figure 7.3) so you know what the official recommendations are in these types of scenarios.

On the day of the exam, you should be more than prepared if you have taken the advice we just offered and solicited questions from your colleagues based on your samples. Your examiner may begin by asking you which case you want to start with. We recommend picking your strongest one. You will have to go through both cases, but we think it can be a helpful boost of confidence that you can use when you defend your second case.

Make sure to listen carefully to questions and answer specifically what was asked. If a question is unclear, it's okay to ask for clarification. Stick to answering the exact question at hand, and avoid introducing new topics that could lead to additional questioning. This is a defense, but don't get defensive if you are challenged on a particular topic or decision. Don't be afraid to acknowledge when you don't know something—part of being a professional is knowing when you have maxed out your knowledge. You can and should say where you would go to look up that information or how you might find the answer to that question.

Remember the scope and purpose of the exam to help quell your anxiety. The exam is a mark of expertise, but this is not a test of knowing everything there is to know in neuropsychology. As you practice answering questions about your sample, try actually saying the words "In my everyday clinical practice, ..." It will help remind you of the goal of the exam: The examiners want to see how you actually think and operate as a neuropsychologist. The key is to stay composed, recognize that limits will be tested and are a part of your oral defense, and acknowledge when you don't know the answer—but follow this immediately with some thoughts about where you would search to get that information if you don't know the answer (hint: think peer consult, checking with colleagues on one of the neuropsychology listservs, reviewing current literature with an article search, reading up from your library of neuro-psychology texts, and so on).

The Ethics/Professional Issues Portion

It may be tempting to treat this portion of the exam less seriously than the others, but we have it on good authority that people can and do fail based on their performance on this section. We provide here some advice to help you prepare. First, develop a template that you can use when you review the ethics vignette. The template should provide reminders such as the Health Insurance Portability and Accountability Act, key legal issues, principles/standards, and the major sections of the American Psychological Association (2017) Ethics Code. Use this as your guide so you can organize your thoughts systematically rather than calling out ethical violations as you read through the vignettes. This template will help you avoid feeling scattered and overwhelmed and ensure that you are comprehensive in your assessment. There are established processes, policies, and frameworks that you can use to approach consideration of ethical issues in these scenarios. For example, Shane Bush's CORE OPT is an excellent model to work from (for more information on CORE-OPT, see Chapter 1 of *Ethical Practice in Forensic Psychology* [Bush et al., 2019]). Also, think about the processes in your current institution—how are these ethical issues managed? Are there any local or state rules that also influence this?

Similar to fact-finding, it helps to hear how someone approaches this portion of the exam. The Navigating Neuropsychology podcast series has a sample ethical vignette, and we think this is a great illustration of how to work through the process (https://www.navneuro.com/115). Also similar to fact-finding, practice is key. Practice reviewing several ethical vignettes; there are a number of them available on the BRAIN website, and use the template you developed to make sure you are addressing all of the ethical violations. If you find you've missed something during your review, adjust your template so you are on the lookout for it on the next vignette. The more you practice, the more confident and prepared you'll be for this segment of the exam. As you practice, we recommend picking up copies of two more of Shane Bush's books: *Ethical Decision Making in Clinical Neuropsychology* (2018) and *A Casebook of Ethical Challenges in Neuropsychology* (2012). Both are excellent and informative reads.

On the day of the exam, remember to use the template that you prepared as you review the vignette to ensure you don't miss any important ethical issues. Normal test taking tips apply. Read the vignette carefully, and take notes to guide your responses.

Although it's nice to be able to memorize the exact numbering of the APA Ethics Code, it's not necessary. What you should be able to do is readily identify them and why a violation would be problematic. Don't just point out what the person did wrong; articulate what they should have done differently. And no less important than the standards are the principles; these are important to know and include in your responses as well. Cite relevant ethical statutes or related professional statement papers, whenever possible. Also, make sure you are not only identifying overt or obvious ethical violations but also pointing out implied issues—those gray areas that are a little less clear but potentially problematic. Altogether, this demonstrates your ability to think from multiple angles and shows that you can navigate complex ethical situations with a nuanced understanding of the principles involved.

The professional issues section is fairly straightforward. You will likely be asked about your education and training trajectory and about the work you currently do. You could be asked about why you decided to pursue board certification. Reflect in advance on how you currently and how you would like to contribute to the field in some way. What are your strengths and areas of growth in your clinical practice? What are some current trending topics in neuropsychology, and what are your thoughts about them? It doesn't hurt to think about an ethical dilemma that you have faced in your own practice, and how you managed it.

ROADBLOCKS

If you don't pass a portion of the exam, don't get discouraged. Avoid catastrophizing ("I failed . . . what if I never pass this exam? What if I never get board certified?") and labeling ("I didn't pass the written exam—I'm a complete failure."). Try to reframe this experience. It helps to recognize that a not-small number of excellent neuropsychologists have failed at least one step of the board-certification exam. That doesn't make them bad neuropsychologists, and neither would it mean that for you. Do not let yourself hinder your progress forward. The key to success is persistence.

Reach out to your colleagues and your mentors and be willing to be vulnerable as you prepare for the next opportunity to retake the exam. Be methodical and honest as you consider what you may have done on the first try that didn't work, and come up with a plan for how you might address this the next go around. The great thing at this stage is that you have more data at this point—you should have a stronger sense of what areas to shore up and what to address specifically when you are preparing for the next time to take the exam. Lesson learned! Just go ahead and schedule that next exam and get right back up on that horse.

8

Finding a Job

Careers in Neuropsychology

 Before working through activities on this topic, be sure to read through Chapters 6 and 7 of *The Neuropsychologist's Roadmap.*

This chapter is all about finding your first job as a neuropsychologist. Similar to other chapters in this workbook, we provide some practical advice based on the responses from 32 neuropsychologists who review job applications. We will present data from this survey throughout the chapter to help you better understand what they are looking for in their job applicants.

APPLYING TO JOBS

By now, you've become a pro at applications! Like all other steps, applying to jobs involves multiple steps over time, as well as several components that make up the application itself. In this section, we break down and review the application timeline and each of the required application materials.

The Application Timeline

As fast as your internship went by, the postdoctoral fellowship is nearly just as quick. Before you know it, you will be thinking ahead to the end goal of your first job. We've provided a timeline for the application process, including steps for preparing your application materials, submitting, and preparing for and completing job interviews (Figure 8.1). The timeline for this phase is a lot more "it depends" in nature because the timespan during which jobs are

https://doi.org/10.1037/0000448-008
The Neuropsychologist's Workbook: A Hands-On Roadmap to Training and Developing Your Career, by C. Block and S. Hickle

FIGURE 8.1. Job Application and Interview Timeline

	Spring				Summer				Fall/Winter			
	Jan	Feb	Mar	Apr	May	Jun	Jul	Aug	Sep	Oct	Nov	Dec
Consider fit factors							▓	▓	▓	▓	▓	▓
Watch for job openings	█	█	█	█	█	█			▓	▓	▓	▓
Work on application/job talk	█	█							▓	▓	▓	▓
Apply and interview	█	█	█	█	█	█			▓	▓	▓	▓

Legend: ▓ = Fall/Winter of your second year of postdoctoral fellowship
█ = Winter/Spring of your second year of postdoctoral fellowship

advertised and candidates interviewed is quite wide. However, you can use this graphic as a rough guide.

In general, the job search begins in your second year of fellowship. It's conceivable that a few positions may be advertised in the fall, so you should be starting to look around during this period. However, the majority of jobs will be advertised from late February to the summer. This is because most institutions like to complete recruitment of interns and postdoctoral fellows, and once the match dates for internship and fellowship pass, then institutions turn their attention and resources toward recruitment of faculty and staff. Don't fret if it's January of your second year and you still haven't seen lots of job openings being announced! It just hasn't hit its peak quite yet.

Once you've taken the step of preparing and submitting your job application(s), the interview process comes next. Typically, institutions notify applicants of their interest fairly quickly. The interview is then followed by the offer, negotiation, and acceptance. The entire process is often completed by late spring or early summer—just in time for you to start your brand-new job! We've provided more information on the components and steps of this process, but first—like all other steps in your training journey—it is important to consider those fit factors.

Consider Fit Factors

You may recall from other chapters that "fit factors" are those things that you take into consideration when weighing institution versus individual aspects. The same goes for jobs: You want to make sure that it is a good match for you, and the more thought you put into the front end of this process, the greater the likelihood that you find a position that truly matches your needs and interests. Using the blank form found in Table 3.2, try inputting some of your own fit factors and running it through a worksheet. We've provided a sample worksheet so you can see what this might look like in real life (Table 8.1).

TABLE 8.1. Fit Factors (Sample)

Fit factor category	Item and response			Score weights
Job factors	Setting	X	3	Academic medical
			2	Veterans Affairs medical center
			1	Private hospital system
			0	Private practice or public hospital system
	Primary duties	X	2	Clinical, research, and teaching
			1	Clinical and one of the above (I can do teaching)
			0	Clinical only, no opportunity for research or teaching
	Training involvement	X	3	Could train fellows, interns, and practicum students
			2	Could train two of the above
			1	Could train one of the above
			0	No trainees I could supervise
Individual factors	Geographic location	X	3	Northeast
			2	Midwest
			1	Southeast
			0	West Coast or Southwest
	Early-career colleague support	X	2	Multiple other early-career colleagues to relate with
			1	One other early-career colleague to relate with
			0	No early-career colleagues
	Financial benefits	X	2	Part of physician incentive plan + professional funds
			1	Only one of the above
			0	None of the above
	Family	X	3	Spouse can work here, good schools, close to parents
			2	Meets two of the above (close to parents, spouse job)
			1	Only one of the above
			0	None of the above
	Total		14	

Feeling stuck? When it comes to fit factors for jobs, we encourage you to think about the institution versus individual aspects outlined in the following list.

- Primary duties: We find that this one takes some thought, mostly because up until now, you've probably found that you've had a hand in many activities like clinical work, research, teaching, service, advocacy, and more. Which one do you envision for your career? It's okay to enjoy most or all of these, and indeed you've likely been doing most or all of these for years as a trainee. At the level of your career, however, you will need to start homing in on the things you are most passionate about, interested in, and good at.

Yes, neuropsychologists do wear many hats, and it is possible to do a little bit of everything. This is especially true in academic medical centers, where you might be seeing patients and doing research and teaching trainees; but even then, you will find that the bulk of your time is spent on just one or two of these. That may even be necessary for advancement/promotion in academic medicine, which expects you to align with a specific promotion pathway. What do promotion pathways look like? Take a look at Figure 8.2, which outlines some sample pathways you might see at an academic medical institution. In essence, you align yourself with one of these as your primary pathway and use that to guide your activities to move you toward career advancement (most often, service is integrated with the first three—but you can sometimes see it as a distinct, fourth pathway). You can see promotion pathways of various institutions with a web search combining the institution name and "promotion guidelines." Ultimately, the point of all this is to say that you will eventually have to choose a relative emphasis in your day-to-day activities (and knowing your top two in advance may help influence which positions for which you are a good fit).

- Setting: Ideally, your education and training have exposed you to a variety of settings in which neuropsychologists are employed. Take a moment to think about these various experiences and ask yourself some questions. Which populations (e.g., age group, clinical diagnoses, referral type) and work activities (e.g., outpatient assessment, inpatient assessment, intervention, research, teaching, mentoring, administration) have you enjoyed the most? What is it you enjoyed about it (e.g., intellectual rigor, sense of purpose and meaning, collegiality, technician support, flexible schedule, benefits)? Now, which setting best matches these? Academic medical (and by extension, a Department of Psychiatry? Neurology? Rehabilitation Medicine?) or

FIGURE 8.2. Promotional Pathways

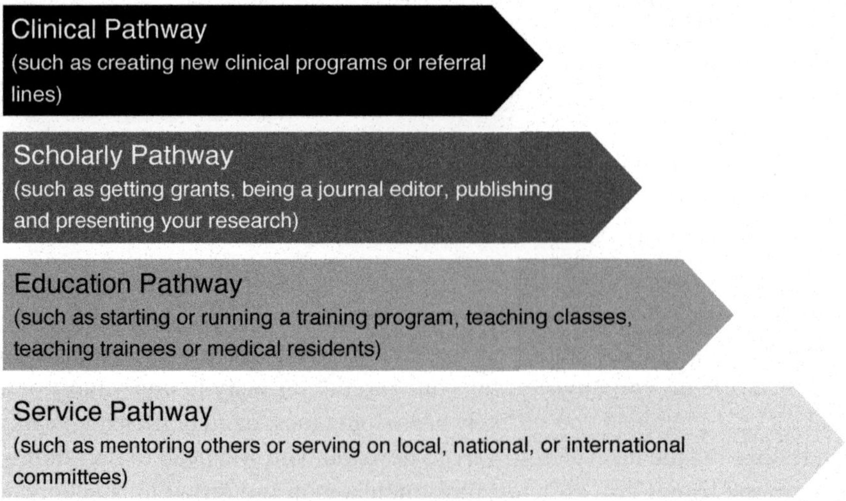

Clinical Pathway
(such as creating new clinical programs or referral lines)

Scholarly Pathway
(such as getting grants, being a journal editor, publishing and presenting your research)

Education Pathway
(such as starting or running a training program, teaching classes, teaching trainees or medical residents)

Service Pathway
(such as mentoring others or serving on local, national, or international committees)

nonacademic medical? Veterans Affairs (VA) Medical Center? Children's Hospital? Private Practice? Academic department at a college or university? Industry? Listen to this webinar by KnowNeuropsychology (https:// knowneuropsych.org/career-pathways) to hear a group of career neuropsychologists discuss careers within academic medical, academic, and VA health care settings.

- Faculty/staff development: Even though you've reached the end of your training journey, the learning doesn't stop there. You will learn as much (or more) in the first 3 years of your first job as you did across internship and postdoctoral fellowship. On top of the expansion of your clinical, research, and teaching skills, you will learn about "The Stuff They Don't Teach You" like billing, coding, productivity, navigating the dynamics and politics of the workplace, leadership, and more (check out Exhibit 8.1 for some resources on this). Continued means for learning and growth are critical, and that comes from faculty/staff development and mentorship programs. When you are at the job interview, ask about how they support the professional development of faculty and staff. Do they pair you with a more senior faculty mentor? Or do they have a more formalized

---

EXHIBIT 8.1

Some Resources on The Stuff They Don't Teach You

The Money and Business Stuff

American Psychological Association billing/coding resources: https://www.apaservices.org/ practice/reimbursement/health-codes/testing
National Academy of Neuropsychology billing/coding webinar: http://tinyurl.com/2w2vd2jj
The Testing Psychologist podcast on billing/coding: http://tinyurl.com/bdf6dk56
IOPC Report Writing Resources: https://iopc.online/report-writing
IOPC Teleneuropsychology webkit: https://iopc.online/teleneuropsychology
"Business in Neuropsychology" (webinar): https://knowneuropsych.org/business-in-neuropsychology
The Business of Neuropsychology (Barisa, 2021)
A Neuropsychologist's Guide to Training Psychometrists (Ghilain, 2021)
The White Coat Investor: A Doctor's Guide to Personal Finance and Investing (Dahle, 2014)
Start Your F.I.R.E.: Financial Independence Retire Early (Redling & Tim, 2020)

The Leadership, Mentorship, and Service Stuff

Society for Clinical Neuropsychology student leadership program: https://scn40.org/ student-leadership-development-program
"The Trainee Leadership Blueprint" (Gooding et al., 2018)
"Mentoring Diverse Trainees" (Sparks & Ellison, 2022)
"Women in Leadership" (Silver et al., 2018)
The Portable Mentor: Expert Guide to a Successful Career in Psychology (Prinstein, 2013)
Supervision in Neuropsychology: Practical, Ethical, and Theoretical Considerations (Bodin et al., 2022)

Note. IOPC = Neuropsychology Interorganizational Practice Committee.

program, such as the FAME program at The Ohio State University (https://medicine.osu.edu/faculty/fame) or the program we have here at Emory University (https://med.emory.edu/about/faculty/faculty-development/career-development/index.html).

• Colleague support: That brings us to our next point: colleague support. It's one thing to be a neuropsychologist embedded in a clinic that has five other neuropsychologists. It's quite another to be a solo neuropsychologist. Early career, or the first 10 years after your doctoral graduation, is an important period in which you benefit from continued support and mentorship—from both early-career peers as well as senior neuropsychologists. These individuals can help you network, invite you to collaborative clinical or research projects, and are a ready source to consult for those difficult situations that eventually arise. This certainly isn't a requirement for a job, and there are other ways to get support such as mentorship programs offered by various neuropsychological societies, but do think about whether this support would be helpful for you.

• Salary: It's okay to admit that salary is an important consideration in which job best suits you. You should be fairly compensated for your time and expertise! We recommend reviewing the neuropsychology salary survey, which is a survey of neuropsychologists within the United States that is completed and published every 5 years (for the most recent data, see Sweet et al., 2021, but be on the lookout for any future publications). This should at least give you a point of departure in determining a fair entry-level salary for something in your part of the country, at your intended type of work setting, and at your level of experience. There are other sources more typically relied on by institutions in determining your salary level, such as the annual data published by the Association of American Medical Colleges or American Association of University Professors, but these are not easily accessible. If the position happens to be a governmental one, state or federal, these are published online and should be easily located with a simple web search. In either case, this information may help you with job selection, and it could certainly be of some benefit during the negotiation process once you receive a job offer.

• Benefits: Get a sense of the benefits a job may offer. These may not always be advertised but could be asked about in the interview process. One thing to consider is if a job has a retirement program; this is something like a 401K or 403B plan, in which you take a small percentage of each paycheck and slowly build savings over time (and you should also look into whether your employer would match contributions by putting in a certain percentage each month). There are also pension-type plans, such as the teacher's retirement fund used by many state academic institutions or Federal Employee Retirement System for VA or other federal employees. Health insurance and disability coverage are certainly also wise to consider. You could also ask about whether the institution qualifies you for public service loan forgiveness or National Institutes of Health loan payback programs; flexibility in the amount of sick leave and paid time off (PTO); flexibility in working from home versus at the office; professional funds to support conference travel or board certification; clinic or research space, furniture, and materials; an allowance for dedicated time during your first year or two in which you can focus on launching your research efforts; and whether there is an institutional incentive or bonus program. Again, you may not always know these things upfront but they are good to consider (and can be included as part of the negotiation process).

- Other factors: There are a plethora of other potential fit factors you could consider, such as geographic location, proximity to your partner's job, quality of the school district for children (if you have them), cost of living, reputation of the institution, the institution allowing you the flexibility for side work (also known as "moonlighting"). We recommend asking your supervisors, mentors, and peers for any others that may not readily come to mind.

THINGS YOU CAN DO NOW

Even if you aren't at the point of looking for jobs yet, there are still things you can do to help prepare in advance. Some of these you may already be doing. First up is research. Throughout your training, some level of scholarship is typically expected. This could range from something as simple as one poster at a local conference all the way up to a publication in an internationally known peer-reviewed journal (and everything in between). In our survey, we asked about the preferred number of publications, oral presentations, and posters that job applicants present with. Survey respondents indicated the following: 6.81 ± 5.45 (range: 0–15) publications, 4.38 ± 4.30 (range: 0–15) oral presentations, and 10.86 ± 8.30 (range: 0–25) posters. If job applications are just a distant speck on the horizon, this could help guide the development of goals around your scholarly output. If job applications are imminent, first of all, don't panic if you are on the low end because you'll notice that the range for each is quite wide. Responses on the higher end tended to come from neuropsychologists within academic departments at universities/colleges and then academic medical settings, although this wasn't exclusively the case, so don't necessarily rule those out if you fall below these averages. However, you may find that it helps guide your remaining time on fellowship. And remember that not all research involves original data collection; there are other options, including using existing datasets, publishing literature reviews or book chapters, or writing up and presenting a case study.

Next is attending conferences. This is a great way to get face time with others to expand your social network (for tips on professional networking, see https://youtu.be/f4hAao-Grdw?si=T6Qxeyj6UxzyzLND). We encourage you to attend any poster sessions, social hours, or receptions at conferences. You could even chat up others in line at the coffee shop within or near the conference hotel. And don't just attend—engage. It might feel weird to approach people you don't know, especially people more senior to you; speaking from the point of people already in their career, however, we can say with certainty that we not only don't mind but enjoy meeting others at conferences. So approach away! But do be thoughtful about it. Come ready with a question or two (people love to talk about themselves). You could ask about the research or clinical work that person is doing, how they are enjoying the conference, or what they are most looking forward to attending while there. Have a 30-second "elevator pitch" ready in which you briefly describe yourself, your training status, what program(s) you are affiliated with, and maybe a little about your clinical and/or research interests. If it makes it a little easier, it's okay to bring someone you know (a friend, a mentor, a supervisor) and have them introduce you to others.

While at the conference, it might help to connect with others about their own job experiences. It should be said that conference socials may not necessarily be the best place to have an in-depth conversation, but they can at least be an initial point of connection to facilitate one-on-one discussion later. When having that discussion, ask questions like the following: What was their job search like? What was the application and interview process like? What sort of things did they negotiate for, and was it successful? How do they like their current position? Did it meet their expectations, or not? What sort of advice would they offer to you?

It also helps to have an online footprint. If someone were to look you up, what would they find? Ideally, you have some sort of professional presence online. This could be as simple as a passive profile on LinkedIn or ResearchGate, or an active presence on social media accounts such as Twitter/X, Facebook, or Instagram. Not only does this help others locate you and get to know you, but they are great avenues for interacting with others to help build your professional network. Recommendations from us: Whichever platform you choose to use, please include a (professional-looking) headshot as well as a brief bio so people can both see and get to know you. If any of said platforms rely on hashtags to link topics, such as #neuropsychology, then use those in your bio to make your profile more likely to show up in search results.

Finally, we recommend perusing existing resources related to careers in neuropsychology. One resource involves the growing number of web-based information content resources dedicated to reviewing careers in neuropsychology (see Exhibit 8.2). Another such resource we've mentioned before is the salary survey, which is an interorganizational survey of neuropsychologists within the United States that is completed every 5 years (Sweet et al., 2021).

LOCATING JOBS

It helps to know all the different places in which you can find jobs. Look at Table 8.2, which breaks these down by type: academic (research), academic (clinical), and nonacademic (clinical). This isn't a comprehensive list, but it does give you some places to get started.

EXHIBIT 8.2

Web-Based Resources on Careers in Neuropsychology

Broad Career Overview

KnowNeuropsychology: https://youtu.be/dKNPOaz4nsU?si=Z_7Xr_Jt7p5QVU_K
Association of Neuropsychology Students and Trainees (SCN): https://www.youtube.com/
   live/PKjnaQG1SkA?si=QulaYC1SkC49k1y6
National Academy of Neuropsychology (members only): http://tinyurl.com/h2kytws6

Specific Careers

Private practice (Early Career Neuropsychologist Committee; SCN): https://youtu.be/
   dKNPOaz4nsU?si=Z_7Xr_Jt7p5QVU_K
Research careers (Early Career Neuropsychologist Committee; SCN): https://youtu.be/
   eaFRUot8fY0?si=s2sDCSM7LqHjJ_Ws

Note. SCN = Society for Clinical Neuropsychology (Division 40 of the American Psychological Association).

TABLE 8.2. Where to Look for Jobs

Type	Place
Academic (Research)	American Psychological Association (PsycCareers): https://www.psyccareers.com
	Association for Psychological Science: https://jobs.psychologicalscience.org
	HigherEd Jobs: https://www.higheredjobs.com/search
	Higher Education Recruitment Consortium: https://main.hercjobs.org/jobs
	The Chronicle of Higher Education: https://jobs.chronicle.com
	PsychJobs Wiki: http://psychjobsearch.wikidot.com
	Society for Neuroscience: https://www.sfn.org/careers
Academic (Clinical)	American Psychological Association (PsycCareers): https://www.psyccareers.com
	American Academy of Clinical Neuropsychology: https://theaacn.org/jobs
	Association of Black Psychologists: https://careercenter.abpsi.org
	International Neuropsychological Society: https://the-ins.org/job-postings
	National Academy of Neuropsychology: https://nanonline.org/jobbank
	Hispanic Neuropsychological Society: https://hnps.org/jobs
	Indeed.com: https://www.indeed.com
Nonacademic (Clinical)	American Psychological Association (PsycCareers): https://www.psyccareers.com
	American Academy of Clinical Neuropsychology: https://theaacn.org/jobs
	Association of Black Psychologists: https://careercenter.abpsi.org
	International Neuropsychological Society: https://the-ins.org/job-postings
	National Academy of Neuropsychology: https://nanonline.org/jobbank
	Hispanic Neuropsychological Society: https://hnps.org/jobs
	Indeed.com: https://www.indeed.com
	Association of Black Psychologists: https://careercenter.abpsi.org
	U.S. Federal Government/Veterans Administration Jobs: https://www.usajobs.gov

If you are looking for a purely academic position related to neuropsychology, then you'll want to head over to the PsychJobs wiki, a repository of academic positions that is updated annually (http://psychjobsearch.wikidot.com). Positions are broken down by area of specialization, and we suggest that those interested in neuropsychology look specifically at the categories of clinical/counseling, cognitive, or neuroscience. There are a multitude of other online repositories to find academic positions, which we've included in Table 8.2. Just to make sure you are covering all bases, however, we recommend that you also periodically scan the job boards hosted by many of the major neuropsychological organization websites including the American Academy of Clinical Neuropsychology (AACN), International Neuropsychological Society (INS), National Academy of Neuropsychology (NAN), and Hispanic Neuropsychological Society (HNS).

If you are looking for a primarily clinical position related to neuropsychology, the mainstays would include those major neuropsychological organization websites: AACN, INS, NAN, and HNS. These are where many academic medical positions are posted, but you will also often see positions advertised for private, public, rehabilitation, or children's hospitals as well as private practice settings. If you are considering going the federal service route (e.g., VA hospital, active duty, or contractor), then a good place to look would be on the USA Jobs website (https://www.usajobs.gov). We also recommend including a third-party search engine in your scouting, such as Indeed.com. This is because many large medical centers use physician recruiters to manage job postings, and these individuals are not familiar enough with neuropsychology to know to advertise on neuropsychological organizational websites; hence, these positions often end up being advertised in other places you wouldn't think to check.

Aside from these resources, there are some other ways that you can supplement your job search. If you are not already a member of listservs such as NPSYCH or those sponsored by major neuropsychological organizations, then we recommend you start joining! After the online repositories listed above, listservs are probably the next most common way to advertise positions. Some less common, but potentially still fruitful, means of looking for jobs come through looking at any job boards that are physically located at various conferences (usually next to or near the registration desk), word-of-mouth, or even by cold emailing. We recommend a blended approach that involves web searches, listservs, and keeping your ear to the ground.

APPLYING TO JOBS

In terms of the number of jobs to which you should apply, our survey respondents suggested an average of 5 to 10 positions. That might sound like a lot, but putting the application together for jobs is not all that different from the postdoctoral fellowship. Your application packet will contain a cover letter, curriculum vitae, and letters of recommendation. There may even be a request for de-identified sample reports. There are a few points of difference worth noting, however. Let's break that down a little further by diving into each section.

Cover Letter

Similar to other levels of training, the application for jobs does require a cover letter. Up until now, cover letters have tended to be structured around fit factors versus areas of need and growth. We think that cover letters for job applications are slightly different in structure, instead using separate paragraphs to highlight your work and accomplishments across different arenas. We have outlined our suggested structure in the following list, but you can of course shift paragraph order based on what you want to emphasize to match the nature of the position.

- Opening paragraph: Introduce yourself and your current position; state your intention to apply to X institution.

- Second paragraph: Detail your clinical interests and training and how those match (or add to) the advertised position. You could consider highlighting a few other things here like how your training was adherent to neuropsychology training guidelines or was supervised by board-certified neuropsychologists.

- Third paragraph: Detail your scholarly interests and training and how those match (or add to) the advertised position. Don't be afraid to toot your horn on any scholarly achievements, noting things like journal or grant review experience, grants, your number of publications (and whether any are first author), in which journals you've published, personal research metrics (see p. 236 of *The Neuropsychologist's Roadmap*; Block, 2021), number of presentations, whether they were oral versus poster, and where your work was presented.

- Fourth paragraph: Here, you could add information on anything else you want to highlight. This could include things such as teaching experience (and, if relevant, any teaching practices or outcomes), awards or honors, or professional service.

- Closing paragraph: Always finish up by expressing gratitude for the reviewers' time and attention, and add a statement about being available should they have any further questions.

Regardless of the structure you choose to adopt, be sure that your cover letter is on professional letterhead and does not exceed two pages. Be firm and confident, and present yourself as a potential colleague, not a student.

Update Your Curriculum Vitae

In our survey, all respondents indicated that they require a curriculum vitae (CV) as part of the job application. By now, you should have a well-rounded CV.

Follow the advice outlined in Chapters 3 (especially Exhibit 3.2 and Table 3.5), 4, and 5 of this workbook to make sure that your CV is well organized and contains all relevant sections to someone at your level.

De-Identified Sample Reports

Similar to fellowship applications, job applications can require the addition of one or more de-identified sample reports as part of your packet. Unlike fellowship applications, however, this isn't very common. Only 21% of our survey respondents indicated that they require this as part of the job application. Nonetheless, you should prepare just in case. When it comes to reports, we asked respondents to rank which aspects they ranked more highly than others. In order of most to least valued were conceptualization, that the case related to a neurologic population, writing quality, test battery, recommendations, and case complexity. We hope this helps guide your selection of reports that best demonstrate your conceptualization skills. As with fellowship reports, review all reports at least once with an eye to de-identification alone. Check your report against standards outlined by the U.S. Department of Health and Human Services (2024; https://bit.ly/3IFVSSI), and be sure to have your supervisor review and approve.

Representative Publications

For more academically oriented or research-focused positions, you may also be asked to include three to five representative publications. Work with your supervisor(s) or mentor to select these. Ideally, these entail original research, were published in well-regarded peer-reviewed journals, and feature you as first author. As a set, they should tie together and reflect the core theme of your research. For example, if you are seeking to be a neuropsychologist in an Alzheimer's disease research center, then you would want to include representative publications related to Alzheimer's, dementia, or related issues.

Letters of Recommendation

Job applications require three letters, ideally from neuropsychologists who know you well. Good people to ask might be a clinical supervisor or dissertation chair from graduate school, your internship director or supervisor(s), and your fellowship director or supervisor(s). Similar to the preceding CV section, we encourage you to follow the advice of Chapters 3 (especially Table 3.7), 4, and 5 of this workbook to review advice on this application component. Providing letter writers with a packet of information is again helpful, although at this level, we would also suggest including the following for each position to which you apply: (a) the institution/department to which you are applying, (b) the title and rank of the job to which you are applying, (c) email and physical mailing address of the institution/department to which you are applying, and (d) deadline.

INTERVIEWING AT JOBS

Before the job interview, make sure you do at least one mock interview with a supervisor or mentor. This is good practice for you in exuding professionalism and responding well to questions, but your "interviewer" can also help catch any distracting verbal or nonverbal habits.

When you do receive an interview offer, know that it often occurs in two parts. The first part is a briefer "meet-and-greet," usually by phone or virtual platform, in which you get to introduce yourself as well as get to know more about the institution, position, and your potential future colleagues. The main purpose of this first part is to determine whether there is enough fit to progress to the second, in-person interview.

In-person interviews can range from 1 to 2 days. They can be exciting and informative, if a bit tiring because the days are long and busy. The institution will likely take care of your travel and hotel accommodations, and you are often treated to meals during the interview process. During business hours, you are meeting with lots of different people. Most likely you will meet the department and/or division chair as well as higher level administrative people (e.g., business operations manager, vice chair for clinical affairs, and so on). You will certainly meet with the faculty and staff, and perhaps even some current trainees if they are available. There is typically a campus or institutional tour as well.

For your interviews, bring one full copy of your application just in case someone requests a copy of your CV, de-identified report, or representative publications. You will likely not be asked for these, but it's a good idea to come prepared. We also suggest bringing a notepad because it's permissible to take notes throughout as you will (and should) be asking a lot of questions. We have provided some sample interview questions in Exhibit 8.3, organized by domain. Just as in previous interviews, it's fine to pose the same questions to different people you meet in the interview. From our survey respondents, here are some additional questions that they recommended: (a) What is your department's track record of promotion of assistant professors in the past 10 years? (b) What are the administrative and service expectations of your junior faculty? (c) What supports are in place for my first 3 years as I am developing my teaching and research (e.g., reduced teaching load, summary salary support)? (d) On which metrics are faculty evaluated, and how are they weighed against each other? (e) What factors have differentiated people who have been successful versus unsuccessful here? (f) What is the expected class load of new faculty? Are there any courses that they are typically expected to teach?

We asked our survey respondents which factors they believed were the most important in considering job applicants during the interview process. In order from most to least important, results were (a) general fit with program, (b) quality of the applicant's responses, (c) professional appearance and attire, (d) quality of the job talk, and (e) applicant seeming well prepared. Perhaps

---

EXHIBIT 8.3

Sample Interview Questions

Sample Clinical Questions

What is the typical schedule/hours for faculty here, and is there flexibility in that?

Do faculty moonlight outside of regular clinical patients? If so, how?

What are the most common referral sources, referral questions, and patient populations for neuropsychological assessment on this rotation?

How are patients scheduled here? Is it a dedicated scheduler, or central scheduling?

What types of test batteries do you typically do here? Is there flexibility in that? How are new tests ordered?

Do faculty do their own testing, or do you use trainees or psychometrists?

When it comes to neuropsychological report writing, can you tell me about the typical length and structure of your own reports? Are providers here on a shared template, or does each approach reports differently?

What kinds of opportunities are available for multidisciplinary work or consultation?

Tell me about the billing process and resources here. Is there a billing department? Who handles precertification/authorization?

What is the clinical productivity expectation here, and what model does your institution use (e.g., based on relative value units, clinic utilization, dollar amount billed vs. collected, or a private practice-type model)?

Sample Education/Training Questions

What psychology/neuropsychology training programs are supported by this institution? How has that changed over the years?

Would I be able to supervise trainees? If so, how do faculty typically handle this?

Would I be involved in teaching or training medical students, interns, residents, or fellows? If so, how?

Is there a case conference or other clinic didactic?

Are there any departmental or medical school/hospital didactics? Are these typically attended in-person or remotely?

Are faculty involved in any institutional, local, regional, national, or international education/training organizational work or leadership?

Sample Research Questions

What resources are available to support starting and maintaining a line of research?

Are there any ongoing research opportunities with which I can get involved?

Are there any internal mechanisms for facilitating research mentorship or collaborations?

How does the institution support early career researchers specifically?

Does the institution sponsor any internal research funding, such as an internal K award program?

EXHIBIT 8.3

Sample Interview Questions *(Continued)*

Sample Institutional Questions

Does the institution require board certification to be completed within a specific period of time? How does the institution support faculty seeking board certification?

What is the professional climate at your institution? Do you interface often (and well) with other medical or psychology specialties?

What is the promotion pathway system here at this institution? Do you have a promotion and tenure guidelines document I could look at?

Does the institution have an internal faculty development/mentoring program? How do you support faculty in moving toward promotion?

What does the institution do to support early-career faculty specifically?

What does the institution do to support faculty who are diverse and/or those from non-traditional backgrounds specifically?

Are there any anticipated institutional or leadership changes coming?

How is the current department/division chair's leadership style?

Are professional funds provided by the institution, and if so, what? (e.g., purchasing and renewing organizational memberships, supporting conference attendance, renewing board certification, renewing journal subscriptions, funds for teaching materials such as books or brain models, funds for clinic or lab space/equipment, office furniture)

Does the institution have an incentive program or other bonus structure? (e.g., sign-on bonus, retention bonus, bonus for completing board certification)

Sample Other Questions

Tell me what it was like getting licensed in this state. Anything I should know in advance?

What has it been like living in (city name)?

When you moved here, were moving costs covered upfront or reimbursed?

Are faculty allowed to moonlight here? Is there an institutional noncompete clause?

Are you offered any professional funds? What does that look like?

What is the work–life balance like here?

---

not surprisingly, similar to other chapters, we see that fit has once again risen to the top of the list!

As far as what questions you may be asked, be ready to discuss the specific reasons for your interest in the institution and why you believe them to be a match for you. Be ready to answer questions about your clinical experience and preferred practice (e.g., what populations do you enjoy most? What test battery do you prefer? Report style and length? What is your typical report turnaround time?). Also, be ready to discuss research (e.g., What are your interests? What was your dissertation topic? What about any publications and presentations? What are your proposed future research plans?) and teaching, education, and mentoring (e.g., Do you have any interest in supervising trainees, and have you supervised trainees before? What is your supervision approach/style? What is your experience in teaching formal coursework versus case conferences or grand rounds?). Some institutions, such as the VA medical system, require performance-based interview questions (for examples, we direct the reader to U.S. Department of Veterans Affairs, 2018). Regardless of question type, however, keep your answers clear, concise, and informative. And don't be afraid to highlight your accomplishments and qualifications! This is not the time to be shy. Toot that horn.

Job Talk

The job talk is a presentation that you give to your prospective employer as a part of your in-person interview. Typically, the talk ranges from 30 to 45 minutes, followed by a 15-minute question-and-answer portion. The audience for your talk will certainly include the other faculty you'd be working with, but could also include other faculty and staff, the division and/or department chair, and perhaps even some trainees. Not all these individuals may be in your specialty, so keep this in mind when constructing and delivering your presentation.

Now, what exactly you discuss will be up to you and the institution at which you are interviewing. In fact, this is a great question to ask before going to the interview: "For my job talk, would you prefer it to be research or clinical in nature, or a combination of the two?" More academically oriented positions will likely prefer that first option, whereas academic–medical or more clinically oriented settings may open it up to the other two options.

If your job talk is research focused, what the institution is looking for is to get a sense of your research competency and productivity via review of your past research efforts as well as your short- and long-term research plans, including how you anticipate starting and growing your lab, taking your research ideas into the future, intended dissemination efforts in publications and at conferences, and plans to seek funding. If your talk is clinically focused, you may instead wish to present an interesting (and de-identified) case you saw within your clinic while on postdoctoral fellowship. You should plan to walk attendees through your case: presenting history, working hypotheses, behavioral observations, results, final conceptualization and recommendations, and a little extra contextual information about the final diagnosis. Often, we as neuropsychologists pursue research that is informed by our clinical work, so a combination talk of this nature can also be well received (and highlight your accomplishments in both areas).

We cannot stress enough the importance of the job talk during the interview process. Your talk can really show "you" at work: your presence, confidence, professionalism, planning and organizational abilities, oral communication skills, teaching skills, time management skills, and ability to think on the spot during the question-and-answer portion. Many candidates at this point look excellent on paper, so the job talk can be a "make or break" factor during the interview process. We urge you to prepare and practice well in advance.

First, take some time to think back on your line of research or the patients you've seen; do any themes emerge? Think about how this presentation tells the story of you through your work. In the meantime, we encourage you to attend a job talk or two (if possible) so you can see what one looks like and how candidates handle questions. Prior to the talk itself, make sure you do a practice run or two with your supervisor or professional mentor—and be sure to have someone time you as well as ask some questions. This will ensure that you are more confident and better prepared on the day of your talk. As far as the talk itself, in Table 8.3, we have shared some of the more important do's and don'ts to consider.

Note of Appreciation

In contrast to other steps in your training journey, it is not only okay but encouraged to send a thank-you letter after you return home from the interview. Email format is fine for this, and use it as an opportunity to briefly reiterate your interest in the position.

TABLE 8.3. Job Talk Tips

Do	Don't
✓ Ask for a 10- to 15-minute prep time beforehand to make sure you are prepared. Make sure you have your slides on a flash drive as well as emailed to yourself (or easily accessible by cloud).	✗ Use too much specialty-specific jargon. Remember: Your audience may not all be neuropsychologists.
✓ Include an outline at the beginning of your talk.	✗ Use overly casual language or filler phrases. Keep it professional.
✓ Be mindful of accessibility guidelines as you design your slide deck: https://www.arl.org/accessibility-guidelines-for-powerpoint-presentations.	✗ Overly rely on notes or absent-mindedly play with them as you speak; this can be distracting to your audience.
✓ Use clear and succinct headers	✗ While moving around the room a little is good, too much back-and-forth can also be distracting to your audience.
✓ Keep it to three or four brief bullet points per slide, using shorter and more straightforward sentences.	✗ Play with your hair or jewelry. Again, distracting.
✓ Speak loudly and clearly.	✗ Be too text-heavy; this creates more work (and increases visual fatigue) on the part of the audience.
✓ Use nonverbals effectively (i.e., good eye contact, smile, appropriate gesturing).	✗ Use lots of different colors, fonts, and other embellishments. You want your presentation to highlight you and your accomplishments. Keep it neat and clean.
✓ Develop supplementary slides, just in case someone has more nuanced questions about your data.	✗ If you do a case presentation, don't accidentally reveal patient information. Make sure everything is de-identified to HIPAA standards.

Note. HIPAA = Health Insurance Portability and Accountability Act.

The Offer

Once the search committee has had a chance to meet and review all job candidates, they should reach out to let you know whether an offer will be forthcoming. This typically happens fairly quickly after the interview—and in some rare instances may even happen at the end of the interview itself. The offer itself will come in the form of a letter, either electronic or paper depending on when the offer is made. It should contain information about the position title, salary, benefits, and terms (e.g., anticipated start date, whether there is a noncompete clause, and so on). Do not, under any circumstances, accept an offer the same day it is made. That offer is yours alone, at least for a limited period of time! You are in the driver's seat. Be cordial and appreciative, and request to schedule a time to discuss the offer and terms—or what is called negotiation.

In Table 8.4, we've provided you with some tips about how to handle the job offer and negotiation when the time comes. We want to underline one particular point: to know and value your worth. You are an accomplished budding neuropsychologist! Don't be afraid to negotiate, and this includes so much more than just your base salary. Revisit the "benefits" bullet in the fit factors section in this chapter, as it outlines several examples of things for which you can negotiate. We can add to that list negotiating your start date (you can request to enjoy a month or two off between end of the postdoctoral fellowship and beginning of the job), work schedule and location (e.g., in-person vs. from home vs. hybrid), reimbursement for moving expenses, sign-on bonus, compensated parking, or even immigration support. There are three possible options in terms of the responses you can review: (a) you will be given what you asked for in entirety; (b) the offer stands as-is, with no changes; and, most likely, (c) they counter-offer with a compromise. Regardless of whether you choose to accept or reject, be gracious and polite.

We want to make special mention of one potential sticky point that your offer might contain: the noncompete clause. This is a statement within your

TABLE 8.4. Offer and Negotiation Tips

Do	Don't
✓ Be cordial and appreciative.	✗ Leave people hanging, it's very poor form. Be timely with all communication.
✓ Request to schedule a time to discuss the offer and terms.	
✓ Seek advice from one or more trusted supervisor(s) or mentor(s).	✗ Take anything personally. This is all just business.
✓ Know and value your worth as a successful budding neuropsychologist. You don't have to just accept an offer at face value.	✗ Negotiate without doing your research. Use the advice in this chapter, and seek out resources (Sweet et al., 2021).
✓ Use competing offers from other institutions to your advantage.	✗ Know when to stop. There are very real financial and logistical limitations, and in reality, not everything can be negotiated.
✓ If any negotiations are made, ask for a revised copy of the offer letter for your records.	✗ Only focus on salary. There are many other things you can negotiate!

contract that would disallow you from the same or similar work, either in full or as a "side hustle." Noncompete clauses can further specify that this limitation exists for a certain period of time (e.g., within 2 years of leaving your job) or within a certain mileage of the city in which you'd be working (e.g., within 100 miles of Neverland). The purpose of the noncompete clause is to protect a company by limiting an employee's (or former employee's) ability to use their resources to benefit themselves or another employer. A good example of this would be doing side work at a private practice in the same city, which could be a no-no depending on what your eventual contract says. This could be another potential point of negotiation, so be sure to read the fine print and fully understand what your offer says. That said, noncompete clauses are not necessarily enforceable across all businesses or even at all in some states, so it behooves you to do a little research to see whether this is applicable to your situation.

Wrapping Up

If you've made it this far, congratulations! Between *The Neuropsychologist's Roadmap* and this workbook, you are now armed with the information you need to snag your first real job as a neuropsychologist. Still, it is worth noting that not all jobs last forever. Sometimes jobs don't work out or your interests or life circumstances change to where the fit is no longer there. This isn't a failure on your part, and in fact you're in good company—many successful neuropsychologists have transitioned between institutions. However, by following the advice we have provided here, ours and that of our survey respondents, you will be in a better position to secure a job that is a good match for you.

CONCLUSIONS

Thank you, dear readers, for allowing us to accompany you on your journey to becoming a neuropsychologist. We hope that you found this workbook eased your way to some extent. The path to neuropsychology can be a lengthy and arduous one, and the end point may not even look the same as when you began. This is because neuropsychology is an ever-evolving field. The way we have practiced in the past is not the way we will likely practice in the future. Part of this entails technological developments in techniques and tools because neuropsychologists are now starting to incorporate telehealth, artificial intelligence, and new computational and statistical methods into the work they do every day. It entails the location in which neuropsychology is practiced as it finds its way into forensic and community arenas. It will also seek to serve more diverse populations. And finally, it will be reshaped by the upcoming Minnesota Guidelines—and in the future, by the next iteration of educational and training standards. We hope future editions of this workbook will help neuropsychologists keep abreast of these.

REFERENCES

American Psychological Association. (2017). *Ethical principles of psychologists and code of conduct* (2002, Amended June 1, 2010, and January 1, 2017). http://www.apa.org/ethics/code/index.aspx

Anderson, V., Northam, E., & Wrennall, J. (2019). *Developmental neuropsychology: A clinical approach* (2nd ed.). Routledge.

Armstrong, K. E., Beebe, D. W., Hilsabeck, R. C., & Kirkwood, M. W. (2019). *Board certification in clinical neuropsychology* (2nd ed.). Oxford University Press.

ASPPB. (2022, January). *EPPP part 2* [Video]. https://cdn.ymaws.com/www.asppb.net/resource/resmgr/eppp_2/eppp2_sample_items_jan_2022.mp4

Barclay Simpson. (2023, November 4). How long do recruiters and employers really spend looking at your CV? https://www.barclaysimpson.com/how-long-do-recruiters-spend-looking-at-cv/

Barisa, M. (2021). *The business of neuropsychology*. Oxford University Press.

Beauchamp, M. H., Peterson, R. L., Ris, M. D., Taylor, H. G., & Yeates, K. O. (Eds.). (2022). *Pediatric neuropsychology: Research, theory, and practice* (3rd ed.). Guilford Press.

Block, C. (Ed.). (2021). *The neuropsychologist's roadmap: A training and career guide*. American Psychological Association.

Blumenfeld, H. (2021). *Neuroanatomy through clinical cases* (3rd ed.). Oxford University Press.

Bodin, D., Stucky, K. J., & Bush, S. S. (2022). *Supervision in neuropsychology: Practical, ethical, and theoretical considerations*. Oxford University Press.

Bordes Edgar, V., Holder, N., Cox, D. R., & Suris, A. (2019). Competence in psychology board certification: Unlike a good wine, it does not get better with age. *Training and Education in Professional Psychology, 13*(4), 264–269. https://doi.org/10.1037/tep0000246

Bush, S. S. (Ed.). (2012). *A casebook of ethical challenges in neuropsychology*. Routledge.

Bush, S. S. (2018). *Ethical decision making in clinical neuropsychology* (2nd ed.). Oxford University Press.

Bush, S. S., Connell, M. A., & Denney, R. L. (2019). *Ethical practice in forensic psychology*. American Psychological Association. https://doi.org/10.1037/11469-000

Clay, R. A. (2012, November). Are you studying too much for the EPPP? *gradPSYCH Magazine*. https://www.apa.org/gradpsych/2012/11/eppp-myths

Dahle, J. M. (2014). *The white coat investor: A doctor's guide to personal finance and investing*. White Coat Investor LLC.

Driskell, L. D., Del Bene, V. A., & Sperling, S. A. (2022). What makes for a competitive fellowship candidate? A survey of clinical neuropsychology postdoctoral training directors. *The Clinical Neuropsychologist, 36*(8), 2041–2060. https://doi.org/10.1080/13854046.2021.1967451

Fujii, D. (2016). *Conducting a culturally informed neuropsychological evaluation*. American Psychological Association. https://doi.org/10.1037/15958-000

Ghilain, C. S. (2021). *A neuropsychologist's guide to training psychometrists: Promoting competence in psychological testing*. Routledge.

Gooding, A., Block, C. K., Brown, D. S., & Sunderaraman, P. (2018). The trainee leadership blueprint: Opportunities, benefits, and a call to action. *The Clinical Neuropsychologist, 32*(2), 263–283. https://doi.org/10.1080/13854046.2017.1386233

Heilman, K. M., & Valenstein, E. (Eds.). (2012). *Clinical neuropsychology* (5th ed.). Oxford University Press.

Hirst, R. B., Thompson, R. C., Markiv, Y., Pilavjian, H., Arastu, S. F., & Markuson, S. M. (2022). A survey of doctoral internships offering clinical neuropsychology training: Updated expectations for competitive applicants. *Archives of Clinical Neuropsychology, 37*(3), 704–721. https://doi.org/10.1093/arclin/acab081

Lezak, M. D., Howieson, D. B., Bigler, E. D., & Tranel, D. (2012). *Neuropsychological assessment* (5th ed.). Oxford University Press.

Macura, Z., & Ameen, E. J. (2021). Factors associated with passing the EPPP on first attempt: Findings from a mixed methods survey of recent test takers. *Training and Education in Professional Psychology, 15*(1), 23–32. https://doi.org/10.1037/tep0000316

Morgan, J. E., Baron, I. S., & Ricker, J. H. (Eds.). (2011). *Casebook of clinical neuropsychology*. Oxford University Press.

Morgan, J. E., & Ricker, J. H. (Eds.). (2018). *Textbook of clinical neuropsychology* (2nd ed.). Routledge.

Norcross, J. C., & Seyette, M. A. (2022). *The insider's guide to graduate programs in clinical and counseling psychology*. Guilford Press.

Parsons, M. W., & Braun, M. M. (Eds.). (2024). *Clinical neuropsychology: A pocket handbook for assessment* (4th ed.). American Psychological Association. https://doi.org/10.1037/0000383-000

Prinstein, M. J. (2013). *The portable mentor: Expert guide to a successful career in psychology* (2nd ed.). Springer.

Redling, D., & Tim, A. (2020). *Start your F.I.R.E. (Financial Independence Retire Early): A modern guide to early retirement*. Rockridge Press.

Schoenberg, M. R., & Scott, J. G. (Eds.). (2011). *The little black book of neuropsychology: A syndrome-based approach*. Springer.

Silver, C. H., Benitez, A., Armstrong, K., & Tussey, C. M. (2018). Voices of leadership: Wisdom from women leaders in neuropsychology. *The Clinical Neuropsychologist, 32*(2), 252–262. https://doi.org/10.1080/13854046.2017.1417484

Sparks, P. J., & Ellison, R. L. (2022). Mentoring in neuropsychology: How theory and practice can support diverse mentees. *Journal of Clinical and Experimental Neuropsychology, 44*(5–6), 337–344. https://doi.org/10.1080/13803395.2022.2125500

Sperling, S. A., Cimino, C. R., Stricker, N. H., Heffelfinger, A. K., Gess, J. L., Osborn, K. E., & Roper, B. L. (2017). Taxonomy for education and training in clinical neuropsychology: Past, present, and future. *Clinical Neuropsychology, 31*(5), 817–828. https://doi.org/10.1080/13854046.2017.1314017

Stucky, K. J., & Bush, S. (2017). *The neuropsychology fact-finding casebook: A training resource.* Oxford University Press.

Stucky, K. J., Kirkwood, M. W., & Donders, J. (2020). *Clinical neuropsychology study guide and board review* (2nd ed.). Oxford University Press.

Sweet, J. J., Klipfel, K. M., Nelson, N. W., & Moberg, P. J. (2021). Professional practices, beliefs, and incomes of U.S. neuropsychologists: The AACN, NAN, SCN 2020 practice and "salary survey." *The Clinical Neuropsychologist, 35*(1), 7–80. https://doi.org/10.1080/13854046.2020.1849803

Tracy, B. (2017). *Eat that frog! 21 great ways to stop procrastination and get more done in less time.* Berrett-Koehler Publishers.

U.S. Department of Health and Human Services. (2024). *Guidance regarding methods for de-identification of protected health information in accordance with the Health Insurance Portability and Accountability Act (HIPAA) Privacy Rule.* https://www.hhs.gov/hipaa/for-professionals/special-topics/de-identification/index.html#:~:text=The%20De-identification%20Standard,-Section%20164.514(a&text=Under%20this%20standard,%20health%20information,used%20to%20identify%20an%20individual

U.S. Department of Veterans Affairs. (2018). *Performance based interviewing (PBI).* https://www.va.gov/pbi/questions.asp

INDEX

ABOUT THE AUTHORS

Cady Block, PhD, ABPP-CN, is a neuropsychologist and associate professor within the Department of Psychiatry and Psychology at the Mayo Clinic in Jacksonville, Florida. Her doctoral, internship, and fellowship training all included emphases in neuropsychology, comprising a PhD in Medical–Clinical Psychology at the University of Alabama at Birmingham, an internship at the University of Oklahoma Health Sciences Center, and a postdoctoral fellowship at Baylor College of Medicine. She previously served as a clinical supervisor for the neuropsychology practicum and internship training programs at The Ohio State University Wexner Medical Center and more recently as training director of the neuropsychology practicum program and departmental internship rotation in the Department of Neurology at Emory University School of Medicine. Dr. Block currently serves as associate training director for the neuropsychology postdoctoral fellowship at Mayo Clinic Florida. She is the editor of *The Neuropsychologist's Roadmap: A Training and Career Guide* and has published numerous peer-reviewed articles related to the training, education, and practice of neuropsychology in national journals. She has also served in a variety of leadership roles in national and international neuropsychological societies, including contributing to the development of the Taxonomy for Education and Training in Clinical Neuropsychology and as an at-large delegate to the more recent Minnesota 2022 Update Conference on Education and Training in Clinical Neuropsychology. She sits on the boards of two international neuropsychology education/training initiatives, KnowNeuropsychology and New2Neuropsychology. In recognition of her work, she is a recipient of several awards including the National Academy of Neuropsychology's Early Career Service Award, the Presidential Citation and Robert A. and Phyllis Levitt Early

Career Awards from the Society for Clinical Neuropsychology, and the Early Career Champion Award and Raymond D. Fowler Award for Outstanding Contribution to the Professional Development of Graduate Students from the American Psychological Association.

Sabrina Hickle, PhD, is a neuropsychologist and practitioner in a private practice. She was previously an assistant professor within the Department of Rehabilitation Medicine at Emory University School of Medicine in Atlanta, Georgia, where she was highly active in Emory's many training programs, including her department's practicum program, internship rotation, and postdoctoral fellowship program. Her doctoral, internship, and fellowship training all included emphases in neuropsychology, comprising a PhD from Georgia State University's joint Clinical Psychology and Neuropsychology & Cognitive and Affective Neuroscience programs, an internship at the VA Boston Healthcare System, and a postdoctoral fellowship at Emory University School of Medicine. Her clinical and research interests are in long-term outcomes from acquired brain injuries (particularly brain tumor, stroke, and traumatic brain injury), as well as the use of network-based neuroimaging methods to better understand the mechanisms through which neurological injuries result in variability in cognitive, emotional, and psychosocial outcomes.